ELEPHANTS
IN YOUR TENT

ELEPHANTS IN YOUR TENT

Spiritual Support as a
Mystic Survives Cancer

Judith Larkin Reno, Ph. D.

Disclaimer: The contents of this book are personal experiences and are not meant as medical advice. These recommendations are no substitute for your medical doctor.

This book was printed in the United States of America.

To order additional copies of this book, contact:
Xlibris Corporation, Philadelphia, PA
1-888-795-4274
www.Xlibris.com
Orders@Xlibris.com
23537

TESTIMONIALS FOR *Elephants in Your Tent*

- "This book is an absolute masterpiece! You will benefit immeasurably—in body, mind, and spirit—from the expert advice of this cancer survivor sharing her success. Indeed, the world will evolve several levels if it follows Dr. Reno's wisdom!"—Dr. Irv Katz, President International University of Professional Studies.
- "Dr. Reno, thank you for sharing your amazing story and the tools you developed for pain control and self-transformation."— Ione Caley, University of Colorado, Cancer Survivor.
- "Dr. Reno is a master of two worlds, transcending life/death duality to embrace True Identity, far beyond earthly confines. In *Elephants in Your Tent*, you will find gifts behind pain, true power under frailty, and an indestructible core beyond the impermanence of life."—Marion Moss Hubbard, Ph. D., author *Work as a Heroic Journey* and *Removing Your Mask*.
- "This book is so incredible! It is truly a lifesaver with the best tools for people going through a difficult time. It is life changing! Everyone experiencing crisis or illness should have this book."—Fern Gorin, Director Life Purpose Institute, San Diego.
- "*Elephants in Your Tent* is an Instruction Manual for getting through times of illness. I cannot convey how very much I resonate with this book."—Marcia Einhorn, Administrative Law Judge.
- "Judith is a ninja, victorious in the battles and vicissitudes of life. Her work is a bounteous fountain of blessings."—Russ Phelps, The Idea Factory, San Diego.
- "Wow! Brilliant!! Judith's powerful insights open the doors of perception."—Kimberly Marooney, author *Angel Blessings* and *Angel Love*.
- "*Elephants* is a gift to humanity, for all who want to embody spirit and live the divine life."—Leonard Laskow, M.D., author *Healing with Love* and *Self Awakening*.

- "Most spiritual healing books provide three notes. Dr. Reno gives us the complete symphony. I pray for many more masterful works from her great heart and pen. Her great passion for God is contagious!"—Carolyn Gross, Director Creative Life Solutions, San Diego, author *Treatable and Beatable: Healing Cancer without Surgery* and *Calm in the Midst of Chaos.*
- "*Elephants in Your Tent* is a roadmap for getting through scary, difficult territory."—Jane Broadwell, Port Administrator, Long Beach.
- "The God Ladder is a tool I use every day. Thank you!"—Survivor.
- "Dr. Reno has a practical, lively approach. She is witty, brilliant, inspired, and joyful. You will find her work enlightening and even fun!"—Donna Apgar, Language Specialist, North Carolina.
- "Dr. Reno's work is a blessing to this world!"—Katy Guard, Director Yoga and Meditation School, San Diego.
- "Dr. Reno opens you to wisdom, love, and miracles!"—Gloria and Barry Blum, Kona's Traveling Jewish Wedding Band.
- "This book is a triumph of the human spirit!"—Satisfied Reader.
- "I am wowed!!! This is such an excellent book with incredible power and depth! It is extremely well-written, with gems on every page. Such a great accomplishment and gift to the world!!!"—Satisfied Reader.
- "**Elephants in Your Tent** is a must-read for anyone who truly wants to reclaim their health, their spirit, and their life."—Judy Saalinger, Ph. D., MFT, author *Fearless Change*, Director Lasting Recovery Substance Abuse Treatment Center.

Other books by Judith Larkin Reno, Ph. D.:

- *Elephants in Your Tent Companion-Book: Spiritual Support to Survive Illness*

- *A Mystic's View of War: Using The God Ladder for Clarity*

- *The God Ladder: Spiritual Initiation for Contemporary Living*

- *Love's Triumph: Child Abuse Recovery with Soul Support*

DEDICATION
Believe in the Goodness!

CONTENTS

ACKNOWLEDGEMENTS

I am deeply grateful to many people who helped me write *Elephants in Your Tent: Spiritual Support as a Mystic Survives Cancer.*

Greatest kudos goes to my husband—beloved, champion, and dearest Bruce—without whom I would not have survived. Bruce cared for me twenty-four hours a day, seven days a week, for three years. He is truly a spiritual man, an embodiment of love and wisdom, and a great playmate! He spent endless hours on the computer with the manuscript, typing, editing, trouble-shooting, and researching. Next to my relationship with God, Bruce is the greatest treasure of my life.

Beloved Revered Guruji, His Holiness Sri Swami Divyananda Saraswatiji Maharaj is another of the greatest treasures of my life. A modern saint from Badrinath in the Indian Himalayas, Guruji was a shining example of God union in daily life. He made his mahasamadhi ascension November 3, 2000, at eighty-nine years old. He taught gratitude to God for all the lessons, even the difficult ones. Mine is a God of love, wisdom, mercy, peace, grace, joy, and endless beauty—in large part due to Guruji's leadership.

Thanks go to my daughters and sons-in-law, Sara and Todd Naidl, and Caitlin and Rob Duin, for their continuous prayers and loving support. Sara called me from Hawaii every day for over a year to spark my life-force. Her powerful, shamanic prayers worked!

Caitlin brought the healing radiance of angels as she solved innumerable problems, including legal matters and finding a recliner. Every day, she read prayers to me from Unity's *Daily Word.* Cait and Rob gave me my grandson Adam, who was born after my first stem-cell transplant. He brought the awesome gift of new life.

You will read about my daughters and Guruji as the elephants begin to dance.

My mother Pauline Graustein was an ongoing support. Her spirit and generosity pulled us through many dark times. My sister Rev. Cariel Quinly delivered energy directly from God's heart. Our bond and deep love made all the difference in my progress. My brother Will Graustein coached me to survive. He said, "Stay strong, Judith." He saw this book before I did. My sister Janice Weisberg sent all the right "power" jewelry that I wore for strength when I had a scary medical procedure. My twelve-year-old nephew Trevor Max Weisberg offered to help "in any way."

My nephew David Sobelman and his wife Angela brought my hilarious, rain-slicker-yellow duck. He quacks when you press his belly. Laughing at this silly, beady-eyed duck gave precious relief from the "hell pains." Angela's powerful healing ministrations went straight to God's ears. My first husband David Larkin was my legal champion. His canasta games helped the rough times go smoother. My Uncle Herb Carter sent jokes and girlhood pictures. My Aunt Elizabeth Cleveland, also a cancer survivor, sent powerful prayers. My Aunt Jean Gavin meditated and prayed for me, as did my Uncle Bob and Aunt Jean Carter and Aunt Audrey Bell.

Rev. Verneice Hammond from San Diego is a world-class healer, Taoist priestess, and dear friend who gave me healing treatments every week. She shook her fist at Death and fought for my life. You will read about her in the chapter on death.

Gordon Burt of Taos, New Mexico is another world-class healer and a shaman who helped me survive against the odds. I have seen Gordon do many miracles. I am honored to know him. I'm grateful for the healing prayers of Gordon and his wife, Cynthia.

Deep thanks to Dr. Glenn Frieder, my gifted chiropractor. A healer of great stature, he never shirked from battle. He always held the highest healing vision for me. His prayers, indomitable spirit, and consecrated life were an ongoing source of renewal.

In addition to family and healers, my friends gave me strength. They walked with me through many dark times, for months on end. Rev. Beverly Nelson was one of the first I'd call when times were darkest. Each time we prayed, I experienced immediate relief and a shift toward hope.

My dear friend Katy Guard is anther mighty prayer-master who walked with me daily in the battle for my life. Her strength and true spiritual warriorship never wavered. She continued to say, "I see you healed"—even through the hopeless times.

Rev. Kimberly Marooney, my beloved friend and another veteran spiritual warrior, was with me every moment in continuous healing prayer. Her *Angel Blessing Cards*, her advanced spiritual initiation, our writing partnership, her rare strength, loyalty, and love were true blessings in my life.

My "Sparkle Plenty" Dr. Lisa Longworth enlisted several Ecuadorian shamans to help me. You'll read about her prayer scroll. She typed the early *Elephant* manuscript and encouraged my writing. She was a constant prayer force. Her love calls, radiant visits, singular artwork, and dazzling spirit helped me build a fortress against the darkness. Lisa literally held my hand through two stem-cell transplants.

Dr. Ruth Kornhauser, Ruti, continuously demonstrated her love— doing errands, helping with the manuscript, praying, and cheering me on. "Maheshwari," Jane Broadwell, drove four hours a week for many months to cook and clean. She was a healing oasis for me. My "Tower of Power" Russ Phelps gave me strength and renewal with his shamanic prayers and healing power. My beloved friend Dr. Inula Martinkatz was always there with a fresh supply of Rumi, Hafiz, love, inspiration, and white roses. Thanks to my dear friend Dr. Irv Katz for his expert hypnosis, a key to my triumph in the stem-cell transplants.

You will read about some of these dear friends who helped me dance with the elephant.

Profound gratitude and love go to my entire Prayer Team. Their strength gave me strength. Their prayers gave me life: Rev. Fern Gorin, Dennis Mesnick, Dr. Helen and Christa Joy Antoniak, Darwin Bree, Dr. Bernie Gunther, Dr. Leonard Laskow, Sally Stryker, Dr. Burt Bialik, Leslie Goldman, Rev. Tera Lamb, Rev. Maggie Benson Smith, Rev. Judi Baxter Wadley, Rev. Kathryn Allen, Rev. Phyllis Rhyner, Rev.

Robert Philley, Rev. Carol Joy Goldstein, Rev. Peter Lowey, Rev. Rich Kirk, John Baty, Daniel and Sarah Larkin, Janet Larkin, Cheryl Larkin, Paul Richter, Julianne Clark, Ayse Underhill, Art and Junko Hopkins, Carolyn Gross, Mouna, Romel Hokanson, Anastasia Weil, Mark and Antra Berger, Rustum Gard, Margaret Leach, Murray Millander, Natasha Stroud, Dr. Judy Saalinger, Carol Linda Vogt, Sandra Lesar, Mile and Nada Vulovich, Capi Johnson, Nonie Bradley, Suzie Walton, Sheri Ittner, Janet Tufford Watson, Rev. Douglas Garland, Rev. Alan and Joan Graustein, Ben Benson, Richard Circuit, Barbara Joyce and Gordon Jones, Bill Watson, Gina Concatelli, Leela Reneene Mowry, Share, Lynne Miller, Laree Blanks, Patricia Blanks, Lynne and Kenny Watkins, Steve and Colleen Blanks, Lee Blanks, Rosie Schaum, Diane Harrison, Sylvana Neal, William Varney, Eric Hedges, Dr. Vivian King, Dr. Mark Krupp, Tom and Mandy Nelson, Tina Stark, and Greg Smith.

Deep thanks to my extraordinary doctors and medical team, all from San Diego County. They were central to my survival. Special thanks to my gifted oncologist Dr. Laurie Frakes for her leadership, skill, and true caring. Thanks to Dr. Robert Brunst for his wisdom, heart, and great expertise. Special thanks to the brilliant Dr. James Mason and the wonderful staff at the Bone Marrow Transplant Unit of Scripps Green Hospital; the great staff at Oceanside's Tri-City Hospital; the staff of San Diego Cancer Center: Tammy Cartmel, Chris Dudero, Barbara Lindstrom, Anita Mason, Amy Isaacs, Jackie Battle, Jennifer Brown, Michele Yount, Theresa Petzinger and Laura Cerda; the staff at Acacia Health Center in Solana Beach: Shivam, Maryann Birchfield, and Vicky Curro; and my excellent physical therapist, Tom Simmons, in Encinitas, California.

In Africa, they say, "It takes a village to raise a child." In my case, it took a "village" to save my life! I am very grateful to every member of my healing village.

The Treasure Lies Deep in the Ocean

—Jelaluddin Rumi

The treasure lies deep in the ocean,
But if it's safety you seek,
It lies back on the shore.

INTRODUCTION

May the energy of your Divine Self inspire you.
May the Light of your Soul direct you.
—Vedic Chant

Sri Ramana Maharshi was one of the greatest Indian saints of all time. He was a twentieth century proponent of the advaita path of Hindu Vedanta. Advaita emphasizes God union through the direct means of continuously asking, "Who am I?" The ultimate, irreducible answer to this question places you face to face with God.

Facing death through a life-threatening disease provides a similar service. It forces you to look beyond personal, earth-bound identities to the unconstructed, pure nature of being. It can bring you to the ultimate enlightenment, God union.

Toward the end of his life, Ramana developed pancreatic cancer which devastated parts of his body and caused great pain. One of his disciples asked, "Master, how can such a great one as you—with full God realization—be attacked by cancer and pain? Why don't you just heal it? Why suffer pain?"

Ramana answered, "The pain is God's will. I am not attached to my physical body or its pain. I live in the deeper Source. God realization is a great energy—sometimes larger than the body can contain or the mind can understand. When an elephant enters your tent . . . many things can happen."

The path to enlightenment is filled with elephants—some raging bulls, some Ganeshas of good luck. Only God knows the value of these elephants. Ramana trusted God's will beyond his own. He trusted the "elephant" process. He believed in the Goodness beyond negative appearances.

If you live long enough, it's guaranteed the elephant will enter your tent in one form or another. What looks like the disease elephant in your tent can be the path to liberation.

Catastrophe is a natural part of life's polarity—swinging from hot to cold, summer to winter, up to down, health to disease, happiness to unhappiness—and back again. The continuous seesaw of reversals is valuable to spiritual growth. Ramana demonstrates that anchoring in God union can provide refuge from life's chaos. He wasn't afraid of the elephant in his tent.

When the elephant enters your tent, I recommend dancing! The great opportunity of dancing with the disease elephant is enlightenment, transcension, and God union. There are many spiritual gifts in the healing dance.

Serious illness creates devastating changes. Opportunities to grieve abound as you lose powers, identity, future, vitality, value, meaning, and motion. You may grieve the loss of friends who can't face disease. You may feel you have lost everything.

Healthy grieving involves resolution. You move through denial, hurt, rage, depression, and sadness to find acceptance. Healthy grieving creates space for new life and new identity.

Enlightenment is a grief experience. You grieve as one illusion after another dies. Each loss expands your inner space. Your identity eventually expands to include God. Disease accelerates the loss of illusions, increasing your opportunity for enlightenment.

It is easy to love God when everything is going well. However, illness tests your relationship with God. How much do you really love God? Do you trust God? Who is your God? Would a loving God hurt you? How do you reconcile trusting God with the losses you experience? What are your values? Does your behavior match your beliefs? Can you surrender your personal agenda to an unseen God's often irrational agenda? How do you avoid bitterness when disease appears to be unjustified? How do you forgive the unforgivable?

As you resolve these powerful questions, your faith deepens. The potential for closeness with God increases. By facing disease, you can discover a richer, more loving spiritual life than you ever imagined.

The roller coaster of modern medicine gives great hope, on some days. Other days, the outlook can be bleak. During serious, long-term illness, you learn the healthy balance of "scientific hopelessness"—the non-attached balance between hope and hopelessness.

Jews in concentration camps during World War II discovered that hope is too painful when it is repeatedly devastated. Hope ran them wild with excitement one day, only to be dashed later. As a healthy defense mechanism, they learned not to identify with hope. Trusting God's will beyond their own, they practiced what I call "holy uncaring."

They avoided extreme emotions, sustaining equanimity in both good and bad news. The tricky part with this detachment skill is not to become bitter, cynical, or shut down—which is simply hopelessness. Equilibrium is an advanced spiritual strength at the core of the illness curriculum.

When you're dancing with a pain elephant, it is easy to lose your balance. You feel alone, living outside the mainstream of life. Your tribe has not experienced intense, radical pain. Few people understand your journey.

Remember however, there is no place you can go in your pain that someone else has not visited. You are not alone. Perhaps, others have made friends with the pain. Perhaps, others have even conquered the pain.

With God as your ally, even cataclysmic events become manageable. You can resolve complex issues of disease, pain, and death. Pope John Paul II said, "Suffering is a gift from God." The disease elephant brings rich spiritual awakening. Don't miss this part!

In my work as a mystic, I chart the inner worlds. I find words that translate mystical experience to earthly understanding. Barry Manilow "writes the songs." As a spiritual cartographer, I make the word-maps to God. I chart the course between the inner and outer worlds.

When I received a diagnosis of two fatal diseases—bone cancer complicated by cryoglobulinemia—I wondered where God would lead me. I wondered if I could describe my healing journey to death and back to life. How do you name the unnamable? How do you describe the indescribable?

Mysticism can be frustrating because the "truths" often contradict each other. Throughout this book, you may notice the paradox of opposites, both stated as true. The mind becomes exasperated trying to make sense of this koan.

However, if you make friends with this contradiction, you expand enough to contain the opposites. Your consciousness grows. Your spirit expands. You open to God's Great Mystery—the Great Unknowing.

Truth extends beyond the province of the mind. Truth spans the many worlds into spiritual terrain. The mind, while good with earth-bound facts, can actually block universal Truth. Spiritual IQ extends far beyond mental IQ.

In *The Doors of Perception*, Aldous Huxley describes the brain as a reductive agent. The brain-mind protects humans from prematurely overloading on the vast supply of cosmic information. Some cosmic energy is too intense for the unawakened consciousness. It can burn-out brain circuitry.

The brain works best within limited earthly realms. However, don't rely on the brain/mind to give you the complete, universal picture. The source of your healing lies far beyond earth's limited time/space box.

Mystical realities require spirit and faith. With spiritual practice, meditation, and prayer, the brain-chemistry changes. Neural pathways shift to accommodate cosmic information without overloading. You step into a completely new range of perception, resource, and healing supply.

Transcending your mind-stuff is a first step to freedom and healing. This transcension is called awakening. Awakening is often a natural by-product of dealing with disease. Catastrophic illness mandates that you construct refuge beyond earth's limited "box."

If you approach God looking only for the rational, you will be greatly disappointed. If you crack through the obstacle of mind, you find new freedom and Truth.

The paradoxes of disease—living while dying, fighting to live while surrendering to death, saying yes to death and yes to life simultaneously—provide great axes to break free from the time/space box. You can transcend worldly limits into God's greater embrace.

The British poet and playwright Coleridge said when you witness a performance presented on stage, you know the stage is not real. You also know the words are not real. However, you suspend your doubt to discover deeper insights. Coleridge called this transcension "the willing suspension of disbelief."

The spiritual study of Truth requires "the willing suspension of disbelief" to escape the tyranny of fact-based, earthly consciousness. Truth extends far beyond the appearance-level of facts. To perceive Truth, you must transcend mind/facts and move into spirit.

Your infinite healing supply resides outside the earthly box. The "monkey-mind," as it is called in the East, is full of illusions and limitations. It can trap you inside earthly reality, sacrificing your access to Infinite Supply.

Dancing with the disease elephant helps you access your power in God Source—beyond the time/space box. You penetrate the hypnotic trance of the monkey-mind and discover your infinite spirit. Through the many trials and tests of disease, you can return to your True Self.

Elephants in Your Tent: Spiritual Support as a Mystic Survives Cancer offers all the spiritual home-remedies that I used to survive catastrophic illness. These are tried-and-true recipes with proven success. I tested each one in the laboratory of my life. This book is filled with hundreds of skills and practical tips for coping with disease and pain.

Pain is invasive. It can destroy your peace of mind. It can even rob your soul if you don't fight back. This book helps you fight back and triumph.

Elephants in Your Tent Companion-Book: Spiritual Support to Survive Illness is a mate to this book. It provides additional skills, exercises, and self-discovery in your dances with elephants. The *Companion-Book* further explores how to connect with angels and nature spirits for healing. Other topics include dealing with posttraumatic stress; self-interview skills (physical, emotional, and mental); emotional sobriety; forgiveness; increasing personal power; cellular installations to increase vital force; holy infusions; spiritual imbeds; sacred indwellings; Soul aerobics; healing prayers, meditations, and poems.

Like bats in your belfry, elephants in your tent can drive you crazy! Don't ignore the elephant in the room. Receive help so you can deal with him. These books give you spiritual support, strength, and renewal to dance with your elephant. They empower you in the healing dance.

My hope is that in your elephant dance, you will break out of the box. I see you dancing into greater freedom and God union. Pain and disease are powerful dance partners. May this book be your dance coach, cheerleading you to dance free!

How to Use This Book

> *If a man carry his own lantern, he need not fear the darkness.*
> —Hasidic

Healing is a mystical journey. It is full of opportunities to engage with God in new and wondrous ways. Enlightenment can be one of the gifts of healing.

Important questions that lead to enlightenment on the healing journey include the following: Who am I? What do I value? Who is my God? What is death? What are my reasons for living?

You may find new answers with each new level of healing. You may reinvent yourself many times as you cycle-up to each new level.

During your healing, you may feel as if you are tangoing with an elephant in your tent. On some days, the elephant may be God. On other days, the elephant looks like disease, death, pain, new life, or your identity. With changing partners and unexpected deep-dips, the dance is never dull!

Think of me as your dance coach. We're a rare and proud breed, those of us who teach elephant dancing. It is a divine dance. We're happy to share our jungle secrets with courageous seekers.

My recommendation when the elephant enters your tent is to dance! Dance! Dance! If one step doesn't work, learn another. Regardless of how riotously your tent flaps, give the elephant a dance to remember! This book offers you great new dance steps. And, it protects your feet!

Elephants in Your Tent fills you with inspiration for living and practical tips for coping. We all have elephants in our tents. Anyone faced with life's quests and questions can benefit from reading this book. It restores your God connection.

Elephants in Your Tent can especially help those dealing with life-threatening disease and pain. Reading aloud gives comfort and quiets the elephant.

This book helps you navigate pain. It is a valuable companion in crisis. It offers multiple levels of healing—physically, emotionally, mentally, and spiritually. You receive both earthly skills and spiritual renewal. Spiritual principles and Truth-training are the foundation of your healing.

Special features include the following:

- **Front line support** to battle catastrophic illness.
- **Skill training**—both practical and spiritual—to manage disease, pain, and fear.
- **Truth-training** to transmute pain to power, the wound to wisdom.
- **Healing slogans** to re-vitalize you. These easy-to-memorize, power-packed phrases are spiritual vitamins!
- **Inspiring quotes, prayers, and meditations** to deliver you to God when the pain takes you away. They help you remember who you are and where your power is.
- **Stories, poems, and first-hand experiences** to encourage you.
- **The God Ladder** to guide you.
- **Vivid, concrete imagery** to penetrate the fog of crisis. Research shows it's easier for a person in trauma to receive help from short, colorful, concrete word-pictures.
- **Humor** to lighten your load and put zip in your dance step.
- **11 interactive segments** to create positive change in your life. Clarity is the first step to manifestation. Writing demands clarity. These interactive sections create tangible growth and self-support.

  - **Inventories, questions, and exercises** to assess and re-value your life.
  - **Journals and logs** to introspect and self-honor.

- **Healing lists** to rescue you on the darkest days. This **unique feature** is specially designed for days when you are in pain and don't have much energy. The lists give you a jolt of high energy—easily accessed and quickly absorbed.
- **Dances with Elephants** for a quick boost and immediate relief. Use these healing lists when you are alone at 3 AM or when no one else can comfort you. These **4 fabulous Elephant Dances** help you keep pace with your pain elephant.

  - **The Brazilian Elephant Samba**—a passionate engagement, done belly-to-belly. Use this dance to *Face Your Fear and Pain,* especially when dealing with needles and medical procedures.
  - **The Boston Elephant Ballet**—elegant choreography. Use this dance to *Distract Your Mind from Pain* and trip the light fantastic.
  - **The Texas Elephant Line-Dance**—a country-style promenade. Use this dance to *Work with Pain* and keep your pain in line.
  - **The Argentinean Elephant Tango**—a fast-moving chase. Use this dance to *Outsmart the Pain,* utilizing your partner's power to your advantage.

- **Use the healing lists as an oracular deck of cards** to receive quick wisdom and guidance. Run your finger along the entries, until one jumps out at you. That's yours! Take its medicine and receive support.
- **A constant, trust-worthy friend** to help you—24/7. You are never alone. You always have a wise mentor and lively cheerleader to support you.
- **Bring this book with you to medical procedures.** Read it in the doctor's waiting room to give you strength.

Elephants in Your Tent engages you with the healing journey from many angles: my healing story, creating allies, building your Soul Council and Prayer Team, metaphysical principles of healing, dealing with pain, your relationship with God, your identity, your will to live, death, and non-judgmentalness.

Elephants in Your Tent presents contradictions, paradoxes, and opposites stated as true. Healing invites you to listen to both your God Self and your earthly self. Each self requires different listening skills. Your God Self has a radically different view from your earthly self. When you realize that both views are correct, you expand your consciousness. You become large enough to embrace the opposites.

There is no single answer in dealing with pain. Some days on my healing journey, I needed a good cry. Other times, I needed to talk with a trusted friend.

At the beginning of my journey, I was afraid to cry, thinking I would never stop. I learned to cry within time limits. As I grew sicker, I became increasingly weak and vulnerable. Crying was no longer an option. It could actually damage my body if I indulged in crying. I needed every ounce of strength to fight for my life. Crying was a luxury I couldn't afford.

The kahuna are wisdom-keepers from Hawaii. They say, "Healing begins when crying ends." I'm not sure it's that simple, since I've found healing through both crying and not crying. The point is to validate yourself and be open to change.

What worked yesterday may not work tomorrow. In healing, you are continuously receiving a new body. You must constantly interview your new body and learn how to serve it.

On days when I was too fragile for emotional release work, I learned to change the channels of my mind. I focused my identity in the God level of my being.

To facilitate the shift of attention, I asked the following pivotal questions: What is passing? What is permanent? What is transient? What is True? What is Real? Where is my power? I learned to take back my power from the pain.

Pain is always transient and ultimately illusion. My True nature is unchanging, eternal, infinite, absolute, perfect, and universal. To deal with pain, I asked myself, "What part of me is untouched by the pain?" I constructed refuge there.

Elephants in Your Tent explores existential and metaphysical issues that naturally arise during a life-threatening disease. Your whole identity may shift as the healing dance takes over your life. You may see life, yourself, God, and other people in a new Light.

There is an old story about three blind wise men. The king asked each one to define an elephant. Each blind man took hold of part of the elephant's body and began describing the elephant. The blind man at the tail said, "An elephant is a moving thing, like a rope that keeps swinging back and forth. Surely an elephant is designed to keep the flies away."

The second blind man touched the elephant's ear. He replied, "Yes, I think you're right, the elephant is designed to keep the flies away, but not by a snake-like device, more by a huge triangular wall that keeps moving back and forth."

The third blind man stood by the elephant's mammoth rib cage. He contributed, "You're absolutely right about the wall-like nature of the elephant. Yes, that's it. The elephant is designed to be a walking, moveable wall."

By the end of the conversation, the king was more confused than ever. He had no idea what an elephant was.

In this story, you can substitute God for the elephant. Most people go around probing divine body parts in an attempt to discover God. We never quite get the whole picture. Of course, God is cagey in this regard, always moving and contradicting himself.

Elephants in Your Tent helps you explore God in his many parts and in his whole, both at rest and in the dance, so you can get the complete picture. This exploration is the healing journey. The gift of working with pain is deeper God union.

Call Out

> *You must remember you are not alone!*
> —Judith Larkin Reno, Ph. D.

In your darkest moments, when the pain steals your identity and disconnects you from your Soul, call out to God. Call your guides, angels, planetary masters, and allies. Reach out. Call for help!

You may not feel that they hear you. But call out with all your might. Your call is not lost. It will come back to you later, when you least expect it.

My Healing Journey

It's easy to love God when there is no pain. Pain deepens
your love for God.
—Judith Larkin Reno, Ph. D.

Sitting in the jaws of death is not a comfortable posture. I remained there in the "hell pains" of advanced bone cancer, complicated by cryoglobulinemia—two fatal diseases—for two years.

Then, by God's grace, prayers of friends and family, my husband's love, my own willingness to fight for life, and excellent medical care, I gradually began the long return to health and freedom from pain. The return took another two years. I battled death and acute pain a total of four years.

During the healing journey, I was hospitalized repeatedly for fifteen months, including two rigorous, life-threatening, stem-cell transplants; eight aggressive chemotherapies; and twelve surgical procedures. I started from extreme adverse conditions, with little hope of survival. I graduated from the second stem-cell treatment in record time and in the top five percent of recoveries.

I learned that healing advances in discrete, quantum leaps. After enormous work, suddenly, as if overnight, new levels of healing open. Nature cannot resist a persistent call. Perseverance is one of the keys to healing.

My healing journey began five years before my emergency hospitalization. During the five years, I went to twelve doctors searching for a diagnosis.

The doctors gave me an assortment of assessments, including the following: allergies, Renaud's disease, shingles, bee stings, infection, dehydration, and electromagnetic imbalance. Some doctors assigned my symptoms of exhaustion to menopause, over-work, or stress. I later learned that my form of bone cancer is very rare, which made it difficult for doctors to diagnose.

During the five-year search for a diagnosis, it was easy to get lost in the maze of medical posturing, conjecture, and hypothesizing. The medical language sounded like legalese, as if it were intentionally designed to obfuscate. Often there were four names for the same medicine: the name the doctors used, the name the nurses used, the commercial name, and the cheaper generic brand name at the pharmacy. Insurance companies talked in an additional, separate language!

Billings were often impossible to follow. One time, in frustration, I called the accounting office of a local medical lab and asked if anyone there could explain the way the system worked. The answer was, "No. We don't even know how it works!"

Before I could evaluate each doctor and move on, it took months of blood tests and assessments. During my five-year search, the pain and exhaustion progressively increased. I passed my fifty-sixth birthday, barely able to function, thinking to myself that I would not see fifty-seven.

It was crazy-making not to have a diagnosis. I looked healthy. I exercised daily, ate right, got plenty of rest, and meditated. My personality was out-going. My energy presented to the world as positive and enthusiastic. I loved my work teaching, counseling, and writing. I hiked in the mountains with my husband. I played my violin in the local symphony.

Who would believe me if I said, "I think I have cancer." There was a giant incongruity between the pain I felt inside and the way my life looked from the outside. Without a diagnosis, I was in No Man's Land.

Chronic pain wears you down psychologically. If it weren't for a lifetime of metaphysical training, I wonder how I would have survived.

I had been a spiritual teacher for thirty years. I had studied and taught widely, including Buddhism, Hinduism, Taoism, Islam, Christianity, Judaism, American Indian shamanism, mysticism, and contemporary New Thought. I traveled the globe studying mystical traditions. Meditation was the foundation of my daily living. Spiritual training was my sustenance.

I loved my work. With a Ph. D. in Psychology and my unique mystical training, my counseling practice offered a special blend of psychospiritual healing. I was skilled at helping clients sort through the inner worlds of the psyche, altered states of consciousness, past lives, the Soul, dreams, and time-travel. It was fun to empower clients with discovery of their own inner realities, identities, and talents.

I also loved my work mentoring students. I had founded Gateway Community Church and Gateway University for the study of higher consciousness in the early 1980's. I loved opening dimensional doorways for students. Catalyzing their natural power and gifts gave me joy. I especially enjoyed training interfaith ministers.

As a mystic and spiritual cartographer, my work was to chart the vast inner worlds. I brought back words to identify the evanescent, subjective, inner planes of reality. I created maps of uncharted realms. Constructing a bridge between inner and outer realities, I awakened consciousness. Students became aware of their deep knowing.

My mystical skills helped me survive my dance with the cancer elephant. I spent months floating among the death bardos, not knowing if I would live or die. My spiritual training gave me a larger perspective—beyond physical life. My relationship with God gave me strength, supply, and refuge to face the challenges of the healing journey.

No wonder the doctors had difficulty diagnosing my case. My symptoms were bizarre. I could wake from a regular night's sleep with four dislocated ribs, a dislocated shoulder, dislocated back, neck, and TMJ. My chiropractor's comment was, "You look like you've been in a car wreck! What happened?"

I frequently experienced "bone balloons," as I termed them. The doctors had never seen them and had no name for them. My knuckles and joints suddenly swelled several times normal size, creating painful paralysis. Luckily, the tests showed I didn't have arthritis—just "bone balloons."

I couldn't sit at my desk for longer than thirty minutes since my feet mottled purple and developed frostbite symptoms—a profound, deep cold down to the bone, that only resolved by a hot bath. My feet were so sensitive, the pressure of bed sheets was unbearable. I eventually designed a foot cradle, with the bedding suspended above my feet, so I could sleep at night. To deal with cold sensitivity, I wore sheepskin *Ugg* boots with layers of heavy clothing in eighty-five-degree weather!

The pain resembled shingles, where billions of long, searing hot needles penetrated my mid-section and legs, accompanied by an unreachable itch. If I scratched the area, the itch and rash multiplied. I was constantly drained by the unbearable itch and burning.

The areas of inflammation eventually became covered with a black necrotic crust, like burned marshmallow. They looked as if gangrene had set in. Indeed, I almost lost a toe to the cryoglobulinemia.

The slightest touch to any body part was excruciatingly painful. Even turning on the light switch became impossible during pain bouts. In addition to these acute symptoms, I experienced chronic ache—the way you ache all over with the flu. I felt black and blue—beat-up inside and out.

My immune system was worn down. I developed allergies I never dreamed existed, such as an allergy to the radiation from my computer monitor. I was allergic to grass, dust, and wind—among hundreds of other allergens. I couldn't sit on the back patio due to allergies. I had acute chemical and environmental sensitivities.

Daily living was strategically exhausting. The perfumes in most commonly used commercial products—such as shampoos, hand creams, and soaps—created serious allergic responses. If someone sneezed in the super market three aisles over, I could contract a life-threatening flu or pneumonia. Leaving my home became a risky ordeal.

With all these symptoms, none of the doctors could provide a diagnosis. What do you tell people if you have no diagnosis and yet you are sporadically too weak to participate in events? You schedule events, and then have to cancel at the last minute, depending on the energy level of the day. You live in a crazy-making, split world where the outside and inside realities don't match.

Until you get a good diagnosis, you can't get good treatment. Finally, I found the right doctor—and not a moment too soon. Within days, I was admitted to the hospital with emergency hemorrhaging.

Without the correct diagnosis, I would have died. I was hospitalized seven times in the next fifteen months, most of them on an emergency basis. All of them were life-threatening situations.

After receiving my first very aggressive chemotherapy, I was extremely weak. My legs went out from under me as I sat down. I fractured a vertebra and dislocated a second one, increasing my immobilization. Now, with a broken back, osteoporosis, and bone cancer, I was bed-ridden for many months.

Muscles begin to atrophy within twenty-four hours of not using them. In the "Flat World" of the bed, simple movements were nearly impossible for me. I was too weak to hold the telephone receiver. I couldn't even hold a hair brush!

I lived in the extraordinarily fragile realm of the "glass people," in constant danger of breaking. The tiniest movement could dislocate or even break another bone. "Slowly she moved" became my new motto!

It was over a year before I could begin the years of physical therapy necessary to rebuild my strength. I had to relearn to walk, dress, sit in a chair, open sliding doors, and ride sitting-up in a car.

For many months after diagnosis, the prognosis was not hopeful. We thought in terms of days and weeks of life expectancy. I was semicomatose, hovering between life and death.

I remembered the Tibetan Buddhist's description of moving through the bardos, going toward death. With each vibratory shift moving into the Clear White Light, you drop another layer of protective earthly armor provided by a healthy body. As you die, you become increasingly sensitive. It's like not having any skin to protect you. Negative words or emotions become exaggerated—even tangibly dangerous, like hot daggers or bludgeons assaulting your body.

I was as defenseless and vulnerable as a newborn baby. The tiniest emotional upset shocked and buffeted me. I appreciated my years of meditation. I used mystical skills to create inner stability and weather the stormy sea of energies.

My spirit ran back and forth between life and death, trying to assess God's will for me. My prayer was, "I will that Thy will be done." However, I couldn't clearly discern what God wanted me to do, live or die.

I was prepared to die. I had experienced a good life. I had found happiness, married to a wonderful man. My two daughters were happily married. I loved my family and friends. I was happy with my work and recreation. When I reviewed my life to see if it were time to leave, there was nothing left undone. My desires were fulfilled.

I saw that if I died, there was a place for me on the other side. I could study and teach. However, as I observed the inner worlds, I realized the people I loved were still in the land of the living. There was more love for me in the outer world.

My Inner Guides said, "You have worked hard in this incarnation. You have been a spiritual warrior, experiencing many spiritual initiations. If you are to live now, it will be to enjoy the harvest of your work. Life always has its ups and downs, but you have mastered the major lessons of your Soul Contract. If you stay now, it will be to enjoy."

The Guides went on to say, "You have an Open Key, a choice point. Sometimes death is not optional. Occasionally, there is a choice. In your situation, it's up to you to decide if you will live or die.

"Although you are prepared to die, your destiny does not require that you die at this moment. Your illness was necessary. It helped many people to grow on many levels, including you.

"If you decide to live, it will be difficult. You will have to fight your way back to health. However, you are accustomed to warriorship. You have lived a life of discipline, integrity, and introspection. You have the tools. If you desire to live, you may."

Receiving this information lifted the veil of confusion. Having clarity, I began the long journey back to health. My spirit became highly focused, like an adamantine diamond—first above my body, then inside my body, then inside every cell of my body. My spirit voraciously magnetized the vital force to live.

My body was an empty shell. I filled it with life. The part of me that is God knew all the techniques for bringing me back from death's door. God created me at birth and every day of my healthy life. He could surely do it again!

All of my life I had been a health food proponent. I took few medications, not even aspirin. However, my inner guidance now was to follow the doctors' prescriptions. "God works through the medicines as well as health foods," my Guides said.

My body was limp and lifeless. The wreckage was enormous. When I surveyed the clean-up work I had to do to get well, I felt like Ingrid Bergman in the movie *Inn of the Sixth Happiness.* When she first arrives in China as a missionary, she faces renovating a decrepit, old, tumbledown building. It looks like a pile of rubble. Her task is transforming it into a habitable shelter.

The lumber is lifeless, gray, and dry—packed with years of dirt and dust. It's difficult imagining how she can transform such chaotic ugliness into a thriving business. However, through steady perseverance, she makes her dream come true.

Determined to live, I confronted disease one night in a terrifying nightmare. It would have been a funny Halloween cliché, if it had not felt so real. The disease appeared in the form of a gigantic bloody eyeball that wanted to devour me.

Gathering all my energy, I shouted at the horrifying enemy, "You can't have me! Get out of my way!" I grew enormous and stepped on the hungry, voracious invader. I squashed it into oblivion.

The nightmare was a precious victory. My psyche had clearly portrayed the disease as a vividly defined, concrete enemy. That focusing work required great clarity and will. Unless I could see the enemy, how could I fight it to heal myself?

My will to live had polarized my consciousness into a life-and-death struggle. The nightmare portrayed my battle. Once I engaged the enemy in the nightmare, the dream battle was easy. I remembered important skills of lucid dreaming:

- Identify dream enemies and allies.
- Always win in a dream battle.
- Call on dream allies to help you.
- Claim your infinite power from God Source.
- Transform dream reality from negative to positive.
- Keep rescripting the dream until you reach perfection.
- Accept only perfection.

Much like the dream world, earthly reality is in a continuous state of flux. It is always changing—deconstructing and reconstructing. My Inner Guides reminded me that the God Self in me is capable of all things—including recreating my earthly form. As in the dream world, I could change my waking dream.

I claimed my Infinite God Supply. After all, God made all of vast cosmic creation. He could certainly remake little me! As in the dream, I clearly visualized the enemy defeated and myself in victory—completely healed.

For inspiration, I remembered India's immortal master Babaji. He is 5,000 years old. He specializes in physical regeneration. He has imbued inert physical form with vital force many times. I called upon him for help.

I also remembered Baird Spalding's five volume series *The Life and Teachings of the Masters of the Far East.* It has many eyewitness accounts of physical regeneration. Some masters created new arms and legs from the stump of a complete amputation. In India, there is an ancient, documented, and respected tradition of physical regeneration.

In the West, the lives of the saints are replete with healing miracles. Jesus revived Lazarus from death. Jesus went on to resurrect from his own death.

I knew that using scientific esoteric skills, I could recreate my waking dream. The victory of my sleeping dream empowered me for the long healing battle that lay ahead.

The integrative sequel to my healing dream came in a subsequent meditation. The disease reappeared. This time it was in the form of a black, sticky tar that invaded my body. The black tar felt like hate. The hate wanted to devour me.

I felt nothing but love for the black stuff. Instead of responding to it with fear or hate, I unified with it. I personified it and spoke to it lovingly saying, "I appreciate your struggle, Black Tar. I know you are working hard to serve me. I can see your suffering. You have come to help awaken me. I am deeply grateful to you."

Feeling compassion, I opened my heart and released sweet love into the ugly tar. The smell of sweet-pea blossoms accompanied the love. The healing love surrounded the black tar with bouquets of kisses.

I was Beauty in the fairy tale, *Beauty and the Beast*. The ugly, black tar was the Beast. I continued to love, love, love the Beast. If my heart had opened any further, I would have turned inside out!

At first, the Beast was defensive, receiving so much love. He became increasingly rude and obnoxious. He tried to provoke me to anger so I would betray him. But I was unmoved. I just kept loving, loving, loving. It felt wonderful to ignore his childish temper tantrums and radiate love.

He saw I was not going to stop loving him. Slowly, gradually, he softened. He dropped his defensive guard and received my love. He became giddy with love, like a dog that enjoys being petted. He soaked up the affection, laughing all the while.

Gradually, he grew smaller. His voice became more distant. I kept pouring love in his direction, until nothing was left of him.

For a few days afterward, I thought I heard his voice laughing. However, he never returned. I knew I had my turf back. My body belonged to me. I was beginning to get well.

No one is guaranteed another day on earth. When you face death through catastrophic illness, you are particularly aware of the precious value of each moment. You live in an intensified awareness of life's beauty.

Through the subsequent months of healing, I became keenly aware of the value of prayer, both my own and others. Because I was hypersensitive from disease debilitation, I could feel when my friends prayed for me.

Each person's prayer energy was distinctive, carrying a different strand of God's luminosity. Lisa's prayers were dazzling, sizzling with vital force, like the name I call her, "Sparkle Plenty." Russ, my "Tower of Power," sent prayers that were strong and steady, with unstoppable healing momentum. Kimberly's prayers were ecstatic and ethereal, anchoring me in the arms of God Spirit.

On days when I floundered, I didn't know if I could continue the fight to live. The healing prayers of my friends and family were tangible life-rafts. I clung to them to stay afloat. Their prayers kept me alive.

To anchor myself in the land of the living, I looked at pictures of my friends. I asked friends to pray for me. I am profoundly grateful to have received so much love and so many healing prayers. It is a rare gift to journey through the death worlds and return back to life.

In addition to the love of family and friends, some unusual spiritual champions fought for my life. In "Verneice Fights Death for Me," you will meet Verneice Hammond, who is a world-class healer and lifetime friend. She stood in Death's Doorway, shaking her fist at Death saying, "She is ours! You're not taking her!" She literally brought me back from Death's Door.

You will also meet my daughters, Sara and Cait. Sara is a young Hawaiian kahuna woman. In "Find the Healing Path," you will see her fight for my life. In "Sunshine Jump-Starts My Life" she brings me healing dreams.

Caitlin prayed for me everyday with her husband Rob. Their call for life was so strong they brought my first grandchild Adam to help me stay on earth. In "The Four-Armed Human Hug," you will feel their healing energy.

Two days before my emergency hospital admission due to hemorrhaging, I took spiritual initiation with my beloved Guruji. You will meet Guruji—and perhaps part of yourself—in "Guruji Shows Me Myself." Swami Divyananda Saraswati Maharaj was an eighty-eight year old saint from the Himalayas. I was blessed to study with him for a number of years before my initiation.

I wanted assurance that he was a "real" saint before creating an official Soul commitment with him. Spiritual teachers who offered more platform flash and charisma than actual spiritual substance had disappointed me many times. Through the years with Guruji, I gratefully realized that God sent me a true spiritual master. I feel privileged to have known Guruji. He was central to renewing my spirit. He gave me strength in the fight to live.

Having taken vows of poverty and celibacy, Guruji wore the orange robe of the renunciate. He became a monk through the Hindu "pope" of Western India. Guruji's teacher was His Holiness Sri Jagat (World) Guru Shankaracharya (Pope) Ryaji Sri Abinov (Unique) Satchitananda Teerth (Saint) Swamiji Maharaj of Dwark, the Western Pontificate of India.

Prior to monastic training, Guruji received a Masters Degree in Physics. He also became a Doctor of Naturopathy. He was well educated and articulate. For a renunciate and monk, he was amazingly savvy to the ways of secular society.

Guruji was Mahatma Gandhi's right-hand man. He went to jail with Gandhi and was with Gandhi when he died. For many years as a monk, Guruji lived on the streets of India helping the poor and sleeping on the ground with nothing but a blanket.

After Gandhi died, Guruji took a vow of seclusion and lived in the Himalayan Mountains at 13,000 feet elevation. One hundred feet of snow piled on his rooftop in the winter. His hut was just wide enough for a sleeping cot. He meditated there for forty years, until he received inner guidance to go into the world and share his saintly wisdom.

I had spent a good part of my life chasing Godmen around the world. I was passionate to deepen my understanding of spirituality. Most often, I was disappointed by men who were mesmerizing public performers. However, they didn't live the spiritual teachings in private life.

Guruji was a pleasant surprise. The congruity of his public teaching and his private living reflected his integrity. Guruji delivered the spiritual goods. He was a true saint. He was the most pure, holy man I have ever known.

I was close to death, just days before emergency hospitalization, when I reached out to Guruji for spiritual initiation. Since he continuously traveled around the world lecturing and serving disciples, I felt lucky he was in San Diego when I needed him.

He walked with me every step of the way through my illness. It was uncanny how he called when I needed him. Each time I experienced a major traumatic shock, within minutes the phone rang with Guruji's call. He said exactly what I needed to hear. He realigned my strength with God. My daily meditations with Guruji gave me sustenance. His holy presence renewed my fight to live.

There were many times when the pain ravaged my concentration so badly I couldn't pray or meditate. Looking at my picture of Guruji, I visualized laying my weary head in his sacred lap—something I would never do in real life, since the disciple is only allowed to touch the master's feet. In my desperation, Guruji gave me safe harbor and refuge in the inner worlds. His loving embrace kept me going. His comfort preserved my sanity.

My dear friend Katy prayed for my survival several hours each day. She sang me to sleep at night over the telephone when the medicines kept me awake. Her spiritual warriorship anchored me in this world. She wouldn't let me give up the fight to live.

My beloved Kimberly walked with me in prayer, night and day. She did energy healings at the hospital during medical procedures. So attuned to my healing, she automatically appeared on my doorstep when I needed emotional processing. Her angelic love messages on my answering service were Soul food that kept me alive.

My friend Bev met my needs before I knew I had them. She welcomed me home from the hospital with a Christmas tree and angel. Her angel music box helped calm my fears and penetrate the fog of pain.

My chiropractor Dr. Glenn Frieder is not only a rare healer, but also a powerful prayer-partner. He set a picture of me on his altar between Buddha and Kuan Yin. When I thanked him for walking beside me in the front lines of the battle to save my life, his instant reply shot back, "There is nowhere I would rather be!"

The ministers I trained organized a prayer tree that continuously sent me prayers and healing strength. Church groups all over the country prayed for me.

Never underestimate the power of prayer in healing! Don't be shy about enlisting prayer support. After all, many spiritual blessings return to your prayer partners for their good works.

I asked everyone I could think of to pray for me. Uncle Herb's church group prayed every week. My dear friend Helen enlisted her nine-year-old daughter, Girl Scouts, nuns, and monasteries all over the country to pray for me. Unity Church in Unity, Missouri receives prayer requests twenty-four hours a day. I'm sure one reason I survived is the many prayers on my behalf.

It was difficult to learn to ask for help and then to open to receive it. As a minister, counselor, and educator, I was a people helper. All my life I focused on giving, not on receiving. There is a certain power in giving and being the savior.

I hadn't realized how saviorship could be a defense against receiving. When you give, you are in control. When you receive, you relinquish control. You are vulnerable. You must open to let the gift inside.

Studies show people would rather give than receive, because of vulnerability and power issues. Acquiring surrender skills was important in my healing.

When I received a "love call" on my answering service, I trained myself to open slowly like a flower to the sun. I inhaled every smidgen of love until I was a tuning fork, vibrating with love from the top of my head to the bottoms of my feet. No prayer or drop of love was wasted on me.

The single person who helped me most in my battle to live was my beloved husband Bruce. I call him Saint Bruce—without exaggeration! He fought for my life every second of every day. He was at my side through every procedure and crisis—without fail.

When there was no reason to wake up in the morning, Bruce was there with his sweet, gentle love. He brightened the days. We laughed at little things—the ants in our ant farm falling off their plastic tree; the teenage bird in the backyard awkwardly learning to sing his song, forgetting half the notes; the neighbor's cat sybaritically sprawling on her back in the sun with her feet straight up in the air.

Bruce carried the full load of the house in addition to taking care of me, since I could barely sit up, let alone walk or clean the house. He did the marketing, cooking, cleaning, laundry, chasing the medical bills, talking with the insurance company, keeping my vast supply of medicines refilled, returning phone calls, doing endless errands, squiring me to appointments, and helping to resolve the many ubiquitous daily crises.

He gave me shots and intravenous medicines at home. He lifted me out of bed for months. He read to me, meditated with me, prayed with me, and found jokes on the Internet for me. His nobility, non-judgmentalness, devotion, selfless giving, strength, and love have seen me through this ordeal. He truly turned darkness to Light.

Bruce and I marveled how every day, even in the darkest times, we laughed. We always had a good time. We asked ourselves, "How is it possible we're having fun in the midst of tragedy?" Somehow, in the grueling demands of each day, we managed to find joy. I count that as God's grace.

People asked me about my healing journey. What happened to you? What did you learn? Who helped you? What helped you? My hope is that this book will answer some of those questions.

Some statistics say 40% of Americans will be diagnosed with cancer. With baby boomers aging, the senior demographic is radically expanding. There is a growing need for spiritual skills to fight catastrophic illness. This book can help you win the battle.

The nearer I came to death, the more I appreciated my relationship with God and the love in my life. My healing journey has given me a deeper commitment to God union.

I am reminded of a poem by Hafiz, the fourteenth century Sufi poet from Persia. Hafiz describes life as a battlefield with warriors falling in every direction in excruciating pain. He encourages you to become a victorious warrior. He says the path to victory is to hold your heart,

> Like a life-giving sun
> Though only if you and God become sweet
> Lovers!

It's easy to believe in God when everything is going smoothly. When nothing is working in your life and you are near death, your relationship with God undergoes the real test. Ultimately, your relationship with God is all you have.

In order to heal, I took apart every wheel, cog, belt, and gear of my God relationship to see what worked and what had value. I threw away a lot of useless machinery. What remains of my God relationship is precious to me.

When the elephant storms your tent, it's good to have someone who has gone before you and who has also danced with a raging, bull elephant. I pass along all my dance steps in hope that the victory dance continues!

ALLIES AND ENEMIES

It is crucial to be diligent about taking care of ourselves,
especially during stressful periods.
—Anonymous

Turn confusion into clarity.
—Judith Larkin Reno, Ph. D.

The Stone Tit Gives No Milk

If you lack clarity, you repeatedly go to the stone tit,
fully expecting milk.
—Judith Larkin Reno, Ph. D.

One definition of insanity is doing the same thing over and over,
expecting a different outcome.
—The Anonymous Work

Here is your **first skill training** in learning to dance with elephants. When you battle chronic pain or disease, you must not only increase your energy, but you must also preserve it. You must not dissipate your energy.

Understanding allies and enemies helps you to maintain your energy for healing. An ally is anything that increases your energy. With an ally, you feel hopeful, happy, positive, strong, and alive. An ally can be an activity, event, memory, attitude, behavior, habit, thought, conversation, person, place, object, time of day, season, food, color, sound, location, clothing, etc. Positivity is a major healing ally.

An enemy is anything that drains you—physically, emotionally, mentally, or spiritually. It can be an activity, event, memory, attitude, behavior, habit, thought, conversation, person, place, object, time of day, season, food, color, sound, location, clothing, etc. Negativity is a major enemy.

There are power feeders and power drainers in life. Become an alert caretaker of your energy. Notice who/what strengthens you and who/what exhausts you. Don't go to a stone tit expecting milk. Cultivate allies. Avoid enemies.

Be ruthlessly honest identifying people who drain you. Often relatives and "loved ones" create holes in your aura. Your energy can leak like a sieve when they come into your day.

You can easily discover if the other person is a drainer. Do you feel more or less energy immediately after he leaves? When you are near the person, do you cover your solar plexus? Do you dread his next visit? If the answer is yes, the person is toxic for you.

You need not confront the other person since confrontation can be exhausting when you are ill. However, it is important that you not see the person. At the very least, minimize visits.

You would not allow Count Dracula or a vampire to drink blood from your jugular vein. Similarly, you must not be around anyone who tires you. Continuously self-interview physically, emotionally, mentally, and spiritually. Notice the moment your energy drops.

Avoid negative people, speech, thoughts, habits, or attitudes. Monitor your own internal negative scripts. Rescript them to positive.

If enemies are unavoidable, fortify and rehearse for interactions to optimize your power. Creating physical space between you and a negative person can provide some protection. Direct the conversation to positive subjects. Minimize your time together. Distract your "enemy" by looking at photos or watching a movie. Stop the visit at the first sign of negativity.

During illness, almost anyone can be draining if the visit continues too long. Consider limiting visits to one hour, so you don't tire yourself.

Beware of a tendency toward unrealistic, over-expectation. This is not the time for heroic indulgence.

It is essential that you conserve your energy. You are not the same person that you were before illness. You must get acquainted with your new self, new tolerances, and new time limits.

Learning to rest is a primary ally in the healing journey. Saying no, nicely, is another ally. As my friend Robert Frey says, "To handle yourself, use your head. To handle others use your heart."

Always go toward the prize of a situation—which is your ally, rather than going away from the pain—which may be the enemy. This simple elephant-dance will keep you from being a victim and turn you into a victor.

Know why you are in a particular place, doing an activity at a given time. Be conscious of what you are doing and why. The "why" is your prize. Go toward your prize.

Avoid fogging-out. Remain clear on right motive and right action. If you notice your energy flagging, your power of "No" is a primary ally. Sometimes, the door is your best ally. Don't stay a moment beyond what is necessary.

Shaman Don Juan taught his student Carlos Castaneda, "Always know where your power is." Your personal power is your ally.

When you enter a room, sense the correct place to sit. What place holds the most power for you? It will vary among people and from one occasion to another. Don't be afraid to change locations until you find your "power spot." Some locations are draining. Others are strengthening. Your power spot is an important ally.

Don Juan said, "Another important ally is clarity. Always know exactly why you are in a certain place and what you plan to do there. What are your motives and your goals? How long do you plan to stay? This knowledge is an ally. Don't dissipate your life energy in meaningless activities."

These are important lessons. They require ruthless honesty and rigorous self-interview. The stakes are high. Your survival is the prize.

It took time before Carlos recognized the importance of clarity regarding his allies and enemies. He continued to go unconscious regarding the right use of his personal power.

One night, he walked into a bar without doing the preliminary discernment work. He forgot to self-interview. He had not clarified why he was there or what he expected from the occasion. Nor had he researched his power spot. Soon a fight broke out. Carlos was seriously injured.

Later, Don Juan reprimanded him saying, "Your time on earth is precious. You must be aware of how, where, and why you are spending it. You must not be reckless or wasteful. You must identify right action. Practice awareness and economy of action. Your life depends on it."

Next time, Carlos understood the value of knowing his allies and his enemies.

Your healing will vastly improve as you strengthen your clarity regarding allies and enemies. Throughout this book, I will give you many healing allies.

Your Allies and Enemies Lists

Have nothing in your homes that you do not know to be useful
and believe to be beautiful.
—William Morris

Keep a log of energy allies and enemies for one week. Identify allies and enemies in both the inner and outer worlds. Inventory what helps or hinders you. Be specific.

Every time your energy grows, name the cause. Give it an ally score 1-10. When your energy depletes, identify the cause. Give it an enemy score minus 1-10.

Name your allies and enemies. In your log, beside each ally and enemy, describe its patterns. Identify the circumstances of your energy boost or depletion. Describe your ally or enemy in detail, including its time of day, people involved, conversation, behaviors, foods, activities, etc.

Cultivate allies. Call positive friends on the phone. Invite them to visit you. Send them love notes and e-mail.

Avoid energy drains. Learn to defend yourself against enemies. Develop strategies to protect yourself.

Pets, plants, family, friends, and spiritual teachers can be powerful healing allies. Other allies in regeneration include exercise, bathing, reading, audio tapes, videos, TV, sunny weather, doctors, nurses, music, chair-dancing, marching, clapping, humming, t'ai chi, massage, and candlelight.

Nature, beauty, humor, and gratitude are fabulous allies in healing. Remember and appreciate your personal powers—speech, sight, hearing, taste, touch, mobility, thought, emotion, and spirit.

Keeping order and beauty in your room brings peace of mind. Choosing uplifting colors for your bed is a healing ally. This book is a primary ally for you in navigating pain and disease. Use it often.

Be greedy in collecting allies. Connect with at least one ally each day. Be ruthless in banishing enemies. You are not in a position to squander your energy.

Write your Allies and Enemies Lists below. Reference your Allies List daily. It will infuse you with positive energy. Use your Allies List during energy depletion or discouragement. Be vigilant to access it during challenges. Add to your Allies and Enemies Lists as new circumstances arise.

Allies List:

_____
_____
_____
_____
_____

Enemies List:

_____
_____
_____
_____
_____

Your Prayer Team

When you love somebody, your eyelashes go up and down and
little stars come out of your eyes.
—Karen, age 7

Create a Prayer Team to support you. Don't be shy. Enlist! Enlist! Enlist! Ask friends and family to pray for you. Ask them to light candles for you. Your Prayer Team is a key to your survival. You cannot overestimate its importance!

Collect pictures of your Prayer Team. Take pictures of them when they visit you. You can take pictures from bed with a minimum of energy. Taking pictures empowers you. If your friends live at a distance, ask them to send their pictures.

Put the photos in your Prayer Team Album, along with inspiring letters, notes, and mementos. Reference your Prayer Team Album daily for added energy.

Don't start believing that your life is your medical care, just because it occupies seven days of your week! Stay connected to your life apart from medical procedures. Reach out to your Prayer Team.

Research shows that those who frequently connect with friends and family have the best recoveries. Make an effort to stay connected with life. Each day throughout my illness, I called one member of my Team. Even if my body was throbbing in pain, I dialed through it. Reaching out is one reason I'm alive today.

Invite love calls. Ask friends to leave love messages on your answering service or e-mail. Their encouraging words fuel your love-tank. They keep you going toward success.

Give love calls. On days when you feel strong, speak of your love. Don't leave it unspoken. As we draw close to death, we see only two things matter: a strong relationship with God and the love in life.

When you have a Prayer Team, you are no longer alone. You have extravagant support. Each member is a gift from God. Don't waste your Prayer Team. Call on it frequently.

List the members of your Prayer Team. Say each name, either silently or aloud. Visualize each face. Look at each member's picture.

Identify the special ray of Light each person brings to your life. What gifts and talents does each one have?

Some members are prayer masters and excellent healers. Each one cares for you deeply. They all pray for your healing. Feel their healing power. Let it in.

Each prayer is a life-raft helping you to stay afloat in the stream of life. **Write the list of your Prayer Team below:**

_____

_____

_____

_____

_____

Your Soul Council

The Sundance enlightened teachers will dance the dream awake.
—Harley Swift Deer, Cherokee Medicine Man

Think of the great beings you admire on the inner planes, such as Jesus, Moses, Mohammed, Buddha, and Archangel Michael. They exist to help you. It is a great honor and delight for them to join your Soul Council. However, you must invite them.

Create a Soul Council composed of planetary masters, guides, angels, gods, goddesses, deities, and higher beings that you love and respect. You may choose from among the many pantheons of the world: Egyptian, Greek, Roman, Hindu, Buddhist, Christian, Islamic, Taoist, Chinese, Norse, Hawaiian, Native American Indian.

Invite Spiritual Hierarchy, patriarchs, prophets, founders of world religions, saints, and heroes to join your Soul Council. Include your higher selves: your Soul and personal God Self. Nature spirits and power animals also make good Soul Council members.

These powerful energy centers of higher intelligence are dedicated to your enlightenment. They will empower you. They will intercede with infinite God Source on your behalf. As you grow close to them, they transmit healing to you.

Collect inspiring pictures of your Soul Council. Meditate on them daily. They emanate palatable rays of wisdom and healing. Every time you look at their picture or think of them, you receive their healing energies. Every time you speak their name, there is an automatic connection.

Develop a personal relationship with each member of your Soul Council. Visit them frequently, just as you would cultivate a friendship on earth.

Talk with your Soul Council continuously throughout the day. Praise them. Express an interest in their work. Tell them about your life. Thank them for the help they give you. Ask them for healing.

Ask for specific guidance. The first thought that enters your mind after your question is their answer. The answer often comes with lightning-fast speed. Your answer may come in images, symbols, thoughts, memories, or synchronicities.

At first, it may seem as if you are imagining the answer. Accept whatever comes. Practice trusting your Soul Council, rather than doubting yourself. Receiving an answer requires openness and trust. The closed fist cannot receive a gift. Listening for answers is a receptive skill.

Asking a question of your Soul Council is an active dynamic. You must clearly focus your mind and deeply desire an answer. Send your question to your Soul Council with your powers of love and will.

Trust and practice. Over time, you will discern the inner voices of your Soul Council. The most important thing is that you call out.

Helping humans is the angels' job. They love it when you call for their help. Ask them to be on your Soul Council. Develop personal relationships with them. Just as with human friends, begin by asking their names. See teams of angels loving and helping you.

Look at your Soul Council on the inner planes often throughout the day. Feel their great power, love, wisdom, intelligence, healing, and support.

Each member of your Soul Council has a different talent and specialty. Some will champion your spiritual warriorship. Others are experts at teaching surrender. Some specialize in compassion, others in forgiveness.

Name each member's specialty. Unify with its essence. Feel it enter your body. The divine energy enlivens every cell of your body. Inhale the energy. Let it in. These are your allies. Let them help you.

Create a symbol for each Soul Council member. For example, a symbol for Jesus might be the cross, for his earthly transcension and resurrection. For Buddha, you might use a lamp since he often said, "Be a lamp unto yourself." Symbols concentrate, focus, and intensify energy.

When you inhale, see the symbol enter your body, anchoring in every atom of your body. See, feel, and know the symbol transferring its healing throughout your body, emotions, mind, and spirit. Experience the healing infusion from your head down to the bottoms of your feet. Feel the healing energy restore you.

Give a flower to each member of your Soul Council in thanks for his help.

Now you have support in both the inner and the outer worlds: your **Prayer Team** on earth and your **Soul Council** on the inner planes.

List the members of your Soul Council below:

_____

_____

_____

_____

SACRED NOW AS ALLY

Practicing the Present

Yesterday is history.
Tomorrow is a mystery.
Today is the gift.
That's why it's called the present.
—Unknown

Here is your **second skill training—practicing the present.** The richness of the present moment is all you ever have. The present is where the finite and infinite intersect. It is where you meet God.

The Sacred Now is where your small, earthly self dissolves into the ineffable vastness of your God Source. Your God Source contains infinite intelligence, healing, and supply. The Sacred Now holds the key to your healing.

To heal pain, you must be present with it. You must see and appraise the enemy to win the pain wars.

Vietnamese Buddhist monk Thich Nhat Hanh says we have been running from the Now for many lives. When we realize we will never find freedom by running, we awaken to Now as all that is. When you dispel the notion that God is somewhere else—voila!—you find God.

Thich Nhat Hanh teaches a charming song to help arrive in the present.

I am home. I have arrived.
In the here and in the now.
I am solid. I am still.
In the ultimate I dwell.

Pain contracts your focus. Spirit expands it. Pain can rob you of the Sacred Now by greedily devouring your attention. Pain can separate you from your infinite God Supply.

If you truly stop in any given moment, there is enough. Anxiety drops away. Lack and limit dissolve.

The Sacred Now is large enough to contain both your pain and God Source. To return to the Sacred Now ask, "What am I identifying with? My Higher Self or my earthly self? Infinite God Supply or limitation? My refuge or my pain?" Expand your consciousness to contain both.

Rather than pushing the river of time—trying to escape the present moment—make Now enough. All that you need is here Now. Allow it to be OK, just as it is—here, Now.

Ram Dass's powerful book *Be Here Now* is a useful mantra. Repeat "Be here now," over and over, throughout the day, to insure that you are present in your life.

When you return to the Sacred Now, internal mind chatter stops. Blessed stillness returns. In *The Power of Now*, Eckhart Tolle says, "The mind resists the Now." Your mind is your biggest enemy to the stillness of Now.

The mind's nature is restless. Addicted to phenomena, it is always busy devouring data, judging, and analyzing. The mind is a stimulation junkie, feeding on movement.

The stillness of the Sacred Now frees you from the mind's dualized quests of good/bad, pleasure/pain, mine/yours, past/future. Unhooking from the mind's tyranny, you stop running. You expand the now to contain God.

Stillness strengthens your spirit. You need spirit to access God's infinite healing supply. To find your spirit, you must outsmart and transcend your mind. While your mind is useful in managing mundane reality, it is an impediment to unifying with God Source.

Tolle points to plants and animals as masters who demonstrate the Sacred Now. He asks, "Would there be a past or a future if only plants and animals existed?" Can you picture an animal wearing a watch!

If you have too much past, your thoughts are riddled with unforgiveness, guilt, and resentment. If you have too much future, you suffer anxiety, stress, and worry. Sometimes, both the past and the future clamor for recognition, simultaneously.

You can return to the eternal Now if you become a clear, still pool of water. Simply become still and witness. Reflect and name both the past and the future—until the Sacred Now returns.

To fight disease, compartmentalize your life. Practice living one moment at a time. Rather than futurizing or reliving past trauma, stay connected with the Sacred Now.

Here are some **skills that return you to the Sacred Now**.

1. Conscious breathing.
2. Relaxing.
3. Stopping.
4. Smiling.
5. Grounding.
6. Centering in God.
7. Naming your experience, physically, emotionally, mentally, and spiritually.

Naming your experience returns you to the present. Develop witnessing skills for your physical, emotional, mental, and spiritual experience. See the chapter on "Pain Management" for "Naming Skills."

As you practice the present, you embrace what is. Rather than running away from life, you bring your God Self to it.

Practicing the present is a path to God. The part of you that is God can handle anything earthly life delivers. Returning to the Sacred Now can decrease your pain and increase your healing.

Practice receiving the gifts of the present.

Conscious Breathing and Relaxing

Take rest; a field that has rested gives a beautiful crop.
—Ovid, Roman Poet

You can return to the Sacred Now by observing your breath. The simple act of following your inhale and exhale restores the eternal present. Watching your inhale and exhale can diminish your pain.

Conscious breathing quiets your mind, unhooking you from past or future problems. Your emotions settle down. Your body calms. Conscious breath-work releases stress and relaxes you—especially during crisis. It is also a powerful tool for cleansing and detoxifying.

You may count your breaths from 1 to 10, starting again after 10. Visualize each number. Adding color to the number strengthens your concentration. Or, you may simply repeat "and one" for each breath.

Don't dissipate your energy through stress. Instead, relax. Relaxing conserves and renews precious energy for healing.

To further relax, monitor your body for tension. Starting at your head, scan down through each section of your body, looking for tight spots that you can release. Scan your head, scalp, face, jaws, forehead—and even your tongue. Relax any tension.

Consciously tense the muscles in your face. Hold the tension. Then release. Feel the stress slide down through your body and out through the bottoms of your feet into Mother Earth. Feel the relaxation enter your body.

Tense and relax your neck, shoulders, chest, and stomach. Tense and relax your abdomen, buttocks, legs, and feet. Use self-talk, inviting the muscles to let go. Say, "Let go and let God support you now."

Inhale relaxation. On the exhale, feel yourself surrendering into the hands of God. The same powerful hands that hold the earth in space, hold you. Surrender into God's care.

Inhale relaxation to every body-part. Exhale tension, toxicity, and stress. Inhale Diamond Sparkle Divine White Light. Exhale darkness.

Do a full-body inhale. Inhale health and vitality throughout your body. Bring relaxation from the top of your head to the bottoms of your feet. Feel, see, and know all the internal organs and glands of your body relaxed, renewed, and revitalized with each breath.

Inhale peace to each body part. See a ray of sparkling God Light dissolving tension. Feel God's healing massage, soothing and smoothing away all the cares of the day. Inhale God's healing Light massage throughout the day.

Through relaxation and conscious breathing, new healing energies circulate in your body. Conscious breathing and relaxation are two powerful allies in your healing journey.

Stopping

Stop the urge to beat time; stop the tendency to focus on the future and forget the intermediate milestones; stop the habit of letting worries and sorrows overtake my life; stop in order to take a breather, to reconsider your needs and refocus your energies, directing them more appropriately.
Chan Huong Nghiem, *The Joyful Path*

Go placidly amid the noise and haste, and remember what peace there may be in silence.
—Anonymous, Church in Baltimore

Where is it we think we are going!
—Judith Larkin Reno, Ph. D.

Stopping can save your life. Remember, an enemy is anything that drains your energy. The mind's endless searching, sorting, shopping, judging, and commenting can be a huge energy drain. Each thought demands energy.

When you are healthy, you can afford the energy loss. However, when you are ill, you need your energy for healing. Simply stopping your mind increases your healing energy.

The monkey-mind tricks you into believing your survival depends on more thinking. Left unattended, the mind chops and fragments you. Then, it will serve you up for lunch!

It is not easy to stop the all-devouring mind. The mind's addiction to phenomena has controlled your life for a long time. You have been running for eons, thinking you are getting somewhere.

However, you can penetrate the monkey-mind's illusions only by stopping. Stopping is the only Rx.

Stopping is where you meet God—in the Sacred Now. Now is the fulcrum of doing and being. It is a magical place of egoless emptiness, surrender, and non-doing.

In the Sacred Now, you let God do your life. Rather than pushing or pulling your life, you are a spectator. In stopping, you simply witness the Sacred Now as it unfolds. You watch your life as it happens.

In his *New Sage Cards*, Dr. Bernie Gunther talks about the "nowhere Now/here." To be Now/here requires risk. You must merge with stillness and nothingness—the Great Nowhere.

Stopping feels like death. However, it is the death of the monkey-mind, ego, or small self. How strange, that as we return to life—to God, to our True nature—we experience it as death.

In modern stress-filled living, healthy instincts are reversed. Going to life feels like death; while going to death through stress feels like life. We identify with illusion rather than Reality, the prison rather than freedom, the pain rather than the eternal Now, the limit rather than the Infinite, the lie rather than the Truth of our nature.

Stopping may feel like a counterintuitive, unnatural act. Actually, it is the path to your True Self. Cultivate stopping as refuge. It is where you return to God in the Sacred Now.

Baby wolves learn from their mothers to walk past meat in a steel trap. The mother strengthens the baby's instinct for Truth and life. By contrast, we humans walk blindly into the trap of the restless mind, fully expecting nourishment. We go to the stone tit expecting milk. We confuse our enemies and allies.

There are few models in life for stopping. Indeed, we get paychecks for doing. There is little validation in Western society for being. Just stopping, dwelling in the stillness, is a revolutionary act!

If illness is threatening your life, to retrieve your power you must learn to stop. Make friends with the stillness. Put space between your thoughts. Value peace and quiet.

Drop your monkey-mind's struggles, scripts, and suffering—your earthly identity. When you stop, they dissolve. You release the burden of your attachments. Surrender into stopping is an awesome moment. It is an irrational leap of faith. After the initial terror, what a relief it is!

Especially in the midst of crisis, learn to stop. Inhale. Exhale. Relax. Smile. Let go. Stop talking, doing, thinking, and moving. Practice being still. Enter the silence.

To strengthen your stopping muscles, see how long you can follow the second hand on the clock, before you think of something else. Practice this exercise until you can stop thinking for five minutes. If your mind is distracted, simply bring it back to task. Be careful not to judge or berate yourself. Just resume concentrating on the second hand. In one-pointed focus, remain Now/here.

As you learn to quiet your mind, you strengthen your divine side. Thich Nhat Hanh recommends that you see every stop sign along the road as the hand of Buddha reaching out. It welcomes you to divine refuge.

Grounding and Centering Questions

Enlightenment is when doing and being unite.
—Judith Larkin Reno, Ph. D.

Fighting pain and disease is war. Be prepared to do battle. You have gathered a powerful armada to win the war. Your healing skills include the following: discerning enemies from allies, practicing the present, conscious breathing, relaxing, and stopping.

Grounding and centering techniques also combat the enemy. These skills strengthen your Sacred Now. They help you choose stillness over chaos and suffering.

Use grounding and centering skills in the following situations:

- When you feel triggered into sudden, exaggerated, run-away, negative emotions.
- When you are overwhelmed and confused.

- When you are numbed out.
- When you are physically exhausted.
- When you feel spacey.

Grounding helps you stay in your body and gather your vital energy. You must be in your body to heal it. Life goes easier when you are grounded. The mental noise in your head stops. The confusion quiets.

Spacing-out is a way of not being here. It dissipates and fragments your attention. It can be hazardous to your health. In the fog of spacing-out, you lose clarity to solve the many problems of disease.

The following Grounding Questions help you do what it takes to stay here. Designed for quick, easy access, let the bold highlights catch your attention. The questions return your focus to the here-and-now. Anchoring you, they help you to name your present moment.

Grounding Questions

- **Who am I?** State your name and other identities. For example, my name is Lola. I am a patient, a mother, a wife, a sister, a daughter. I am a perfect child of a loving God.
- **Where am I?** Identify your specific location. For example, I'm leaning over the bed . . . I'm on the phone.
- **What am I doing?** Describe the act in which you are involved. Be detailed and specific. For example, I'm struggling to find my slippers under the bed . . . I'm praying for the right words to comfort my crying child.
- **Why am I here?** Tell why you are involved in this act. For example, I need my slippers to get the walking exercise around the hospital unit that I promised myself . . . I'm comforting my child because I love him.
- **What is the date?** Stating the date and the day of the week can be very grounding. It returns you to the Now.

These Grounding Questions return you to your body and the present moment. When you are grounded, you automatically access the infinite supply of the Sacred Now.

In addition to the above list, to quickly restore grounding, feel hot coals on the bottoms of your feet. Feel your feet heavy and cemented to the ground. Inhale down into your feet.

Visualize an anchor dropping from the base of your spine into the center of the earth. Inhale deep into the center of the earth connecting with your anchor.

The following questions center you in God. They link you to your infinite healing supply. Combating the insanity of the ravenous, restless monkey-mind, they restore your peaceful trust in God.

The God-centered life is always successful, since God does not make mistakes. When you are centered in God, you trust the one basic Truth: *Perfection is everywhere—always.* You trust the perfection of events, knowing that whatever happens could not be otherwise. Despite negative appearances, you know the Truth of your life's perfection.

To maximize healing, center in your infinite God Supply. Make God your center and you lighten your pain load.

Centering Questions

- **Where is my power?** Your power is always in God, the Source of your being—even though it appears that your power is in doctors, a medical procedure, or the medicine. The Source of all power is God. While doctors and medicines are instruments of God, they are not your True Source.
- **Where is God?** God is here, now—always. Wherever you are, God is. Your God Source is eternal and unchanging. Your God Source has infinite intelligence, healing, and supply. Return to your God Source by stopping, grounding, breathing, relaxing, smiling, naming, and embracing the Sacred Now.
- **Where is my gratitude?** Find your gratitude and you find God. What are you thankful for in the here and now?
- **What am I identified with? My infinite God Source or my limited physical self?** Are you taking your identity from your pain? Learn to see beyond the appearance level of earthly facts. Include God in your Sacred Now.

- **Am I surrendered to God's will?** By letting go of your physical concerns—surrendering them into God's care—you return to the God level of your being. You trust God's will beyond your own. You True-Source from God rather than false-sourcing from external events, pain, or people.
- **Who is in charge?** God is always in charge. Despite external appearances, the Reality is that God is the root cause. God is the source of all events in life. Right action involves surrender to your divine side. It is wisdom to know when to surrender your pain to God. Let God carry it.
- **What is True?** The one basic Truth is *Perfection is everywhere— always*. Affirm divine order in your life rather than lack and limit. Keep turning your situation until you see how it is perfect. Truth centers you in God.
- **How must I change to accept the perfection of my situation?** What is the pain teaching you? What false beliefs must you drop to know your life is perfect, here, now? What negative emotions must you relinquish?
- **Am I judging God and life wrong? Am I judging myself wrong?** Judgment is the opposite of God union. To return to your God center, surrender judgment.
- **What is my goal?** Keep your focus riveted on the reward of your medical treatment rather than on the pain. Focus on what you are gaining, not on what you are losing. Your goal may be to walk, to graduate from the hospital, or even to die with dignity. Keep returning your thoughts to your goal. Keep your mind clear of pain fog. Go toward your goal, rather than away from the pain. Stay centered in your power, rather than in your loss.

Be present in your life. Show up! Use your **Grounding and Centering Questions** frequently to access your limitless God Supply of healing. The Questions restore your power through Truth. Grounding and centering are valuable weapons to fight pain.

When you center in God, you return to True Power. One definition of sin is to be off target. To center in God is to be right on target.

TOOLS FOR HEALING

No one is alone if they've come to believe in a Power greater than themselves.
—Alcoholics Anonymous

Nothing can endure the Light of Truth, except Truth.
—Judith Larkin Reno, Ph. D.

To take appearance for reality is a grievous sin and the cause of all calamities. You are the all-pervading, eternal and infinitely creative awareness—consciousness. All else is local and temporary. Don't forget what you are.
—Sri Nisargadatta, *I Am That*

Krishna's Pearls of Wisdom—Principles That Heal

You'll see it when you believe it.
—Wayne Dyer

Stand in the Light that casts no shadow, the healing Light of Truth.
—Judith Larkin Reno, Ph. D.

Construct refuge in Truth.
—Judith Larkin Reno, Ph. D.

The Hindu deity Krishna had a beautiful string of perfect pearls. He taught his students that if you look into any one pearl, you can see the whole world reflected in it. Every pearl contains the whole.

The following principles are like Krishna's pearls. They connect you to the whole and return you to God union. Even if you don't believe in the principles at first, practice them, and they will work for you.

Krisna's Pearls of Wisdom help you conserve energy for healing. Aligning with Truth is energy efficient. You don't dissipate energy on false beliefs and negative thinking.

Use Krishna's Pearls when you are lost in pain. They connect you with your infinite healing supply. The Pearls return you to your God Source.

This is the beginning of your **Truth training**. Truth is the foundation of your healing skills. Krisna's Pearls of Wisdom are a healing credo. Access them frequently on your journey. Wearing them restores you to your divine nature. They help you remember who you truly are.

Krishna's Pearls of Wisdom

Thoughts

- Energy follows thought.
- Thought is creative.
- Your thoughts create your reality.
- Your thought is as tangible as the furniture in the room.
- Positive thought increases healing energy. Negative thought decreases healing energy.
- Discern negative from positive thoughts. Make no judgments. Just discern.
- Replace negative with positive thoughts.
- Foster positive, elevated, high-energy thoughts that heal you.
- Buddha said, "You are what you think. All that you are arises with your thoughts. With your thoughts, you make your world."

Beliefs

- Your thoughts reveal your underlying beliefs.
- Your beliefs, as well as your thoughts, create your reality.

- Identify positive and negative beliefs behind your thinking.
- False beliefs are negative. They create lack-and-limit thinking. They disconnect you from your infinite God Supply and healing.
- Your beliefs create your thoughts and actions. Your actions create your habits. Your habits create your destiny.
- Your beliefs become your biology.
- Cultivate positive beliefs for healing.
- William James said, "The greatest revolution of our generation is the discovery that human beings, by changing the inner attitudes of their minds, can change the outer aspects of their lives."

Emotions

- Emotions are engines adding power to your thoughts and beliefs. Emotions magnify and intensify your thoughts and beliefs.
- Negative emotions often originate in negative, false beliefs.
- Negative emotions can deplete you.
- For healing, cultivate positive emotions. Resolve negative emotions.

Internal and External Realities

- Your external reality appears in the events of your life. Your internal reality is how you respond to events.
- Your internal reality is more important than your external reality.
- You can't always control your external reality. However, you can control your internal reality.
- Your thoughts, beliefs, and emotions create your internal reality. They also can create your external reality.
- Many additional forces create your external reality. You are an expression of God Source. Both your personal God Self and the impersonal God Source create your external reality. Your Soul Contract before birth creates your external reality. Your body and genes create your external reality. The collective creates your external reality. Time and place create your external reality.

- To create a positive internal reality, change your thoughts, beliefs, and emotions from negative to positive. Find the positive gift in every negative event. When you don't understand events, trust God's plan beyond your own.

Your Soul Contract

- Prior to each incarnation, you choose your Soul Contract in league with God—including life events, people, places, and things.
- Your Soul Contract is based on learned and unlearned lessons from your past lives. It helps you to learn and grow into deeper God union in this life.
- While there are legitimate victims at the physical level, at the Soul level there are no victims—since everyone chooses her Soul Contract.
- There are many possible reasons for choosing pain. It can be a way to awaken to Truth. Pain can also be a sacrificial path serving the collective.
- Great Souls often choose complicated, challenging Soul Contracts.
- If you face catastrophic illness, self-witness the greatness of your Soul in choosing an advanced Soul Contract. Honor the complexity of your life path.

Responsibility

- Your response to life is your response-ability. Your ability to respond is like your money. Spend it wisely.
- You are responsible for both your internal and external realities. You chose your external reality through your Soul Contract. You choose your internal reality every moment with your response to life.
- You can't always create positive events in your life. However, you can always choose a positive response to events.
- You retrieve personal power when you accept responsibility for your life without blaming.

- You have powerful abilities to respond to even negative events. Limitless healing, intelligence, and supply lie within you. They are your birthright.
- You are made in God's image. Infinite God Source is hardwired into your design. Access God Source in your response to life.

Avoid Self-Blame

- If you face a negative situation, avoid self-judgment. Many dynamics create your external reality. Some are beyond the reach of your conscious mind.
- Which "you" created your disease and pain? Your universal God Source? Your personal God Self? Your Soul? Your Soul Contract? The collective? Your mind, thoughts, or beliefs? Your emotions or psychological condition? Your lack of exercise, poor eating, not enough rest, shallow breathing, stress? Your genes?
- Correct as many errors as you can. But don't judge anything wrong. You did the best you could throughout your life, given the information you had at the time. Fix what you can. Leave the rest up to God.
- You did nothing wrong. Pain and disease are part of the human journey. No one gets out of here alive! Saints and gurus die of disease. A large majority die of cancer.
- God doesn't make mistakes. You are God in human form.

Pain and Disease

- Pain and disease are not good or bad. They just are—like passing weather.
- Illness is not a sign of failure. You are not a bad girl/boy if you get sick! God is not punishing you.
- The conscious mind cannot fathom the many reasons for illness—or its many benefits.
- Ancient wisdom honors illness as a way the tribe advances. The ill person performs a sacred service cleansing and transmuting the tribe's negative past—creating a bright new future. The tribe respects the sick person's sacrifice.

- Some spiritual traditions say illness can literally change human DNA to design the new human for the New Wisdom Age ahead.
- Through your healing journey, you may be evolving humankind!

Make No Judgments

- Judgment contains moral charge and vindictive condemnation. Judgmentalness carries a projection of unhealthy shaming.
- Judgmentalness comes from unresolved false-belief or emotional trauma. Unresolved issues polarize perception into right/wrong, black/white, them/us judgmental thinking.
- Judgment traps you in the illusion of earthly duality. It disconnects you from your infinite God Supply.
- Increasing negative karma, judgment binds you to the wheel of reincarnation.
- Judgment blocks your liberation, your healing, and your God union.

Discernment vs. Judgment

- Discernment is naming without blaming. It is an objective assessment, apart from your ego or personal projection.
- Discernment is clear perceiving. It is detached, impersonal, and un-invested.
- Discernment comes from your higher mind and divine bodies in concert. By contrast, judgment comes from your lower mental-body, your critical ego-mind—your monkey-mind.
- Discern, but don't judge yourself, others, life, events, or God.

Witnessing and Naming

- Witness your life as if you are a detached observer. Imagine you are watching the movie of someone else's life. Become a spectator of your life.

- Make no judgments, just discern.
- Name the experiences of your life—physical, emotional, mental, and spiritual. Include both positive and negative experiences.
- Naming is not blaming or judging. Naming is a discernment skill. It is objective witnessing, without excessive emotional charge.
- Naming is reporting the many levels of facts and Truth in your life.
- Facts exist on your earthly levels: physical, emotional, and mental. Truth originates on your divine levels: intuitional, Soul, personal God Self, and impersonal God Source.

Discern Truth from Facts

- Facts reside inside the time/space box of relative, earthly existence. Facts change with time and space. By contrast, Truth originates in the absolute realm of your divine side. It is eternal, infinite, and perfect.
- Truth sets you free. Facts can imprison you.
- Facts make a better servant than master.
- Truth is always positive. Facts can be negative.
- To find Truth, ask What's passing? What's permanent? What's ephemeral? What's eternal?
- Truth unites you with God and healing.
- There is one basic Truth: *Perfection is everywhere—always.* Find the Truth here now. Discover the Truth in every moment.
- External realities are fact-bound until you shine the Light of Truth on them.
- Truth liberates you from suffering and attachment. Truth helps you manage pain. Truth prevents confusing your identity with pain. Truth transmutes negative to positive.
- Standing in Truth, you see beyond the present moment of pain or catastrophe.
- Factual pain is transitory and illusory. Pain always passes.
- Love, wisdom, peace, beauty, praise, gratitude, goodness, and harmony lead you to Truth.

- Truth is healing. Speak Truth to yourself and others. Multiply Truth in your life.
- Rescript negative, limiting, false beliefs into positive affirmations of Truth.
- Positive thinking is not denial or repression of facts. Rather, it honors facts while reframing negative to positive through life-affirming principles of Truth.
- Use positive principles of Truth to detoxify negative life circumstances.
- Ask what is factual? What is True.
- Your healing refuge is Divine Truth.

Your Identity

- Don't confuse your identity with your life!
- Don't confuse your identity with external events, people, places, or things.
- Don't confuse your identity with your pain or disease.
- Don't confuse earthly facts with eternal Truth. Your True Identity cannot be found inside the time/space box of temporal change.
- Your True Identity is in your infinite, eternal God union.
- Find that.

Trust God's Plan for You

- God's plan for your life extends far beyond your earthly understanding. God's plan may differ from your own.
- Surrender your personal plan to God.
- Form an alliance with God. God is your best friend. The God in you is the part of you that will never die, betray, or leave you. Ultimately, God is your only ally.
- Construct refuge in God.
- Everything that happens is part of God's perfect plan. Everything happens for a reason. Everything is for the good, though it may appear negative at first.

- Trust the Goodness underlying external events.
- Great Souls embrace great challenge.

Conflict with Others

- When you are ill, conflict with others is not worth the energy payment.
- Observe the energy in conversations. When it polarizes, back off. Soften your heart. Rephrase from unity and love.
- Harmony is healing. Go up your God Ladder to find it.
- Don't expect others to understand your healing journey. They never have had your experiences.
- When you drop expectation, you drop emotional pain.
- The world is your mirror. Everything outside you reflects something inside you.
- Take responsibility for what belongs to you. Fix what is yours. Surrender the rest to God.
- Keep a soft heart.

The Work

- Discern earthly from divine realities. Learn how to care for both aspects of your being. Firmly anchor your identity in your Higher Self.
- Fight to heal and grow against a backdrop of profound surrender to God's will.
- Don't be trapped by facts. Discern the earthly facts. Then, transcend facts. Move into divine Truth.
- Use your God Ladder to return to your infinite healing supply.
- Cultivate God union.

Reinvent Your God

- If you want to know who your God is, observe your thoughts for twenty-four hours. What you think about most of the time is what you worship. Energy follows thought. Your energy payments of thought, over time, create your God.
- False beliefs about God can keep you in pain.

- In advanced healing, you may want to reinvent your God until you construct a trustworthy God.

Let God In

- Open to receive God's love. It is a tangible experience. It is not a concept or abstraction.
- See, feel, hear, and know God loving you—literally. Feel God's love in your bones, blood, brain, and being. Open the doors and windows of your body, heart, mind, and spirit. Let God in.
- Don't block, squander, waste, ignore, or spill God's love. When is the last time you felt God's love? Do it now. It is here, now.
- Practice feeling God in your body. God loves you through each day's beauty, harmony, peace, love, lessons, growth, and gifts.
- Gratitude is the express elevator to God's heart.
- God's love is healing.

Rejoice!

- Life is a gift.
- There is nothing to do but rejoice and give thanks!
- It's all good, regardless of whether your limited earthly mind can see it.
- Trust the Goodness.

Your God Ladder

No people can be ignorant and free.
—Thomas Jefferson

Spirit is untouched by pain.
—Judith Larkin Reno, Ph. D.

Mom and dad teach baby about her physical anatomy. Conquering new territory, baby proudly points to her elbow. On the day baby discovers her own elbow, everyone rejoices.

Imagine today that you are discovering the full range of your complete spiritual anatomy. It is vastly more complex than your physical body. Think in terms of having 7 bodies, rather than one. You have 7 elbows rather than just one!

Your God Ladder helps you discover your 7 bodies including your 4 divine bodies and your 3 earthly bodies. There are profound differences between your internal, divine equipment and your external, earthly equipment.

Truth and healing originate in your divine side. Your divine equipment transcends earthly limits of time and space. Your **4 divine bodies** include **your impersonal, universal God Source; your personal God Self; your Soul; and your intuitional body.**

Your earthly realm is where facts, illusion, conflict, suffering, and false beliefs reside. Your **3 earthly rungs** include **your mental, emotional, and physical bodies.**

Contrasting with your infinite, eternal, perfect divine side, your earthly side is limited, temporary, and flawed. Different laws govern each of your 7 bodies. Both the limited and unlimited sides of your nature must be honored.

Earthly and divine realms marry through you and your life. For example, I am God having the human experience through Judith. You are God having the human experience through your earthly bodies. Human life is the intersection of the relative and absolute worlds. The finite and infinite join here in the human experience.

The 7 levels of your God Ladder anchor in your physical body through your chakras. Chakras are spinning vortices of intelligent energy that vitalize your life. They download information from God to the 7 domains of your life. Their input shapes your consciousness.

You can loosely identify the **7 rungs of your God Ladder** in your physical body in the following locations:

The God Ladder

- **The 7ᵗʰ rung**—The consciousness of your impersonal, universal, infinite, eternal **God Source** correlates with your **crown chakra,** at the top of your head.
- **The 6ᵗʰ rung**—Your **personal God Self** correlates with your **third eye**, in the center of your forehead.

- **The 5ᵗʰ rung**—Your **Soul** in its active aspect correlates with your **throat chakra**.
- **The 4ᵗʰ rung**—Your **intuition** is the receptive aspect of your Soul. It correlates with your **heart chakra.**
- **The 3ʳᵈ rung**—Your **mental body** correlates with your **solar plexus chakra**.
- **The 2ⁿᵈ rung**—Your **emotional body** correlates with your **mid-abdomen chakra.**
- **The 1ˢᵗ rung**—Your **physical body** consciousness correlates with the root chakra at the **base of your spine**.

These 7 rungs of your God Ladder are instruments of your healing. Each rung contains its own learning agenda, vocabulary of ideas, assignment of meaning, and morality.

Each of your 7 bodies has a different Operating Manual—with different rules for care and maintenance. Think of each domain as a state-specific realm with its own applications, powers, problems, talents, and hazards. There are 7 separate Law Books for your complete anatomy.

Each rung is a loading and transition zone, connecting higher and lower levels of your awareness. Sorting, assessing, and digesting your experience, the rungs translate from one domain to another. They negotiate and mediate various aspects of your consciousness.

Explore and delineate each of your **7 bodies: impersonal God Source, personal God Self, Soul, intuitional, mental, emotional, and physical.** Discover your complete anatomy just as a baby delights in discovering her new body.

Feel the differences at each level. Imagine what each domain is like in terms of sight, sound, taste, touch, and smell. What symbol appears on each rung?

Notice your various levels during the day. From which of the 7 levels do you most frequently operate? Which level is most difficult for you? Which level is easiest?

Your God Ladder helps you access your complete anatomy and all your powers. It gives you perspective and clarity. God Ladder calisthenics strengthen your spirit and your healing.

Your God Source

Forgetfulness of the Self, is the source of all misery.
—Sri Ramana Maharshi

In the self-discovery tour of your God Ladder, focus on the 7th rung—your impersonal, universal God Source—at the top of your head. Your transpersonal chakra links you with your Cosmic Source. It is the part of your consciousness that is God.

God Source is the matrix from which all creation emerges. It is the Source of all that is, was, and ever will be. Your God Source is omnipresent, omniscient, and omnipotent. It is infinite and eternal. Imagine a Source so great that it can create everything in the universe!

You plug into that Source when you return to your 7th rung for healing. Your God Source is the part of you that is almighty. You are capable of miracles!

God Source is the Mind of God, the intelligence of the universe. It contains infinite healing and supply. Your 7th rung is the most important part of your God Ladder equipment!

Think of your God Source as a giant warehouse containing energy essences, which are the building blocks of the universe. This unconstructed, vast, energy potential is so rarefied that there is no form.

At the 7th rung, there is no earthly consciousness. The Great Mystery is ineffable and inscrutable. It extends far beyond your limited earthly view. Trying to understand God Source with your mind is like an ant trying to understand the Internet! You can only access God Source through your spirit which exceeds and transcends your mind.

God reformats at each descending rung of your Ladder. God moves from unconstructed Source at the 7th rung to create your personal God Self, your Soul, your intuition, your mind, your emotions, and your physical body. Each level is God manifesting in different forms.

As spirit descends the God Ladder into matter, each lower rung adds heaviness. At the bottom of your Ladder, God energy reaches its grossest vibration—the tangible, physical world. Earth's gravity attracts unconstructed God energy into earthly form.

Your 7th rung God essence is the part of you that remains unchanged from one lifetime to the next. Your God essence is your I Am presence—the part that never dies.

Your God essence is the indestructible, irreducible, indivisible element in you that perpetually "exists" in God Source. Simultaneously, your God essence localizes in your human equipment for a given lifetime. Despite being opposites, the two realms—the absolute and relative, earthly and divine—coexist in your human journey.

Your God essence is the part of you that remains when everything else dissolves at death. At death, your God essence returns up your God Ladder to God Source for re-deployment to another lifetime or cosmic location.

To find your God essence, ask the following questions: What part of me is irreducible? Who remains after I remove all of my earthly identities? Who am I apart from all the external roles I play in life? Take away wife, mother, sister, teacher, student, traveler, writer, counselor . . . and who am I?

Just as a fish doesn't know it's in water, you can overlook your permanent God essence since it never leaves you. What part of you never leaves? Your God essence is closer than yourself.

What part of you neither comes nor goes? What part was there at birth and will be there after death? What part of you remains during deep, unconscious sleep? What part monitors your life continuously, whether you are awake or asleep?

You can also find your permanent essence by identifying the part of you that was the same at five years old, twenty-five years old, and fifty, etc.

"Find that which you can't lose. And be free!" says the song by Kirtana. Find the place inside that is untouched by pain or change. This is your permanent God essence. It is the part of you that is God Source.

Imagine the immense power of God Source out of which all-that-is emerges. Universes, galaxies, star nurseries, celestial bodies, rivers, mountains, oceans, the furry nations, the feathered ones, the mighty air sylphs, the fire devas, the scaled creatures, the four-leggeds, the insect nations, the stone world, the grass brothers, the Green Man, and the two-leggeds, including your human body and every aspect of your being—all were created from your God Source.

Magnificent and awesome is the power of God Source that lives within you! God Source resides in every atom of your body and every aspect of your being. You contain the infinite power of the universe to create. Think of your potential for healing!

Your Divine Bodies

Everywhere men are born free, but live in chains.
—Rousseau

Your divine bodies include the upper 4 rungs of your God Ladder: impersonal God Source, your personal God Self, your Soul, and your intuition which is the receptive aspect of your Soul.

Moving from impersonal God Source to the 6th rung, discover your personal God Self—anchored in your third-eye chakra. Your God Self focuses infinite Source energy into your individual signature for this life. It is the first rung that resonates with your personal essence. Your God Self is your personal strand of God's luminosity—your presentation of God on earth.

Your personal God Self is the Lord God of your being. It is also your personal repository of universal Truth in a given lifetime. All your ideas, beliefs, and projections about God reside in your 6th rung personal God Self. These ideas change throughout a lifetime.

Your personal God Self holds the blueprint for your perfect design. Restoring you to your perfection, it is a valuable ally in healing. Your God Self is a primary gateway to infinite God Source.

Your 6th rung personal God Self is reachable with your mind. By contrast, impersonal God Source is beyond the reach of your mind. It is unconstructed. Beyond concepts and words, technically, there is no way you can "think about" infinite God Source. Thinking requires a subject and an object.

7th rung, unitive God Source is non-dualized. There is no subject/object distinction. All is one. God Source extends far beyond earthly polarities of time and space, subject and object. To connect with

God Source, you use your spirit which far transcends your dualized mind.

Your 6th rung personal God Self houses your spirit. Your God Self is a safe bridge between familiar earthly life and the vast, inscrutable God Source of your 7th rung. Your God Self translates the incomprehensible Infinite into human understanding. It brings limitless resource into your grasp.

Your God Self can access knowledge of all that is, including all creation and past lives. Your God Self consciously transcends time and space—past, present, and future. With far-memory of human evolution, other planets, and other realities, there is little ignorance in your God Self. Instead, there is the Clear White Light of Truth.

Your God Self embodies the Divine Father. At the 6th rung, you study Truth, the law, detachment, and transcension. You clearly see the differences between eternal Truth and ephemeral facts. You distinguish the Real from the unreal worlds. Your God Self integrates infinite, perfect, absolute domains with earth's limited, relative world.

Coming down the God Ladder, you move into your 5th rung, which is the active dynamic of your Soul. It anchors in your throat chakra. At the 5th rung of your Soul, you demonstrate love/wisdom in the world through right speech, right action, and manifestation.

Love, nurturing, compassion, forgiveness, and wisdom are your Soul's agenda. Radiating Golden Light, your Soul embodies the Divine Mother. Like your God Self, she is a gateway to God Source.

Just as a healthy parent names and validates the child's journey, your Soul identifies and values your experience—as well as you. Go to the embrace of your Soul when you need comfort. An adoring mother, she loves you unconditionally.

The voice of your Soul is always kind—never negative. Nobility, forgiveness, beauty, and joy characterize her. Often, your Soul begins speaking with "Dear Child."

Your Soul translates the Truth of your God Self to your personal life. She brings wisdom to your daily journey.

The Soul's job is to keep track of your Soul Contract—your learning agreement before birth. Assessing your strengths and weaknesses, your Soul Contract for this life is based on past-life achievements. Your Soul Contract clearly delineates what you must learn in this life. As a wise parent, your Soul oversees your education.

Your Soul has both an active and a receptive body. At the 4th rung, your heart chakra is your Soul's receptive instrument. It correlates with your intuitional body. You often hear the "still, small" voice of your Soul through your intuition. You develop conscience and wisdom through the direct-knowing and love of your Soul.

Your intuitional body is a psychic information clearinghouse. Here, you begin receiving non-local knowledge, transcending time and place. Information gathers in your intuitional body from all over the multiverse—far beyond earth's time/space box. Your intuitional body also contains data from past, parallel, and future lives.

Everyone receives this non-local information, though not everyone remembers it. When you evolve through spiritual initiations, you consciously develop your intuitional body and far-memory. You begin to read the Akashic Records of the intuitional realm.

At the 4th rung, your psychic talents emerge, such as the following: clairvoyance, clairaudience, clairsentience, empathy, precognition, intuition, astral information, astral projection, dreams, channeling, psychometry, past-life memory, future memory, time-travel, telepathy, telekinesis, etc.

It's easy to be trapped in the glamours of psychic powers and manifestation skills. Power brings with it the perils of abuse. However, if you use the skills of your intuitional body wisely, under the guidance of your Soul, you can create healing and goodness.

On the ascension arc of your God Ladder, spiritual initiation at the 4th rung blasts you free from earth's time/space box. Your intuitional body opens you to entirely new worlds beyond earthly reality. Your identity radically shifts. You clearly "get" that you are far more than skin-encapsulated consciousness!

On this initial God Ladder tour, we are using the descension arc. Later, in "Journey to the Mind of God," you will become familiar with both the ascension and descension arcs of your God Ladder.

At birth, you descend your God Ladder on the ride into earthly life. You move from spirit into matter. The descension arc digests and integrates divine essences, translating them into your earthly bodies.

At death and during sleep, you ascend your God Ladder. You move from matter into spirit. You also ascend your Ladder during meditation and prayer. On the ascension arc, you access the infinite supply of your God Source and digest your earthly life.

In the course of spiritual evolution, you consciously ascend and descend the God Ladder—moving from your earthly to divine identities and vice versa. In fact, everyone ascends and descends the God Ladder continuously throughout the day. However, most people are unconscious of this natural journey between their divine and earthly bodies.

In conscious healing, you ascend your God Ladder to access infinite healing supply from God Source. Then, you consciously descend to infuse healing into your physical, emotional, and mental bodies. By understanding your God Ladder, you can transform your earthly life.

Your Earthly Bodies

The true conquests, the only ones that leave no regret,
are those that are wrested from ignorance.
—Napoleon Bonaparte

The lower 3 rungs of your God Ladder are your earthly equipment. They include your mental, emotional, and physical bodies.

Continuing to tour your God Ladder, you descend from your intuitional body, to your 3rd rung. Here you shift from divine to earthly reality. You make the descent from spirit into matter. Your mental body loosely correlates with your solar plexus chakra.

Between the 4th and 3rd rungs, you cross the Psychic Barrier. Your Psychic Barrier is a reality threshold. You must penetrate it in the evolution of your consciousness. It holds the secrets of the relative vs. absolute worlds.

On the descension arc during birth, at the Psychic Barrier you move from being a gleam in God's eye into fleshly form. With your birth certificate, you gain access to your lower 3 bodies.

Above the Psychic Barrier, you access the upper realms of your infinite, eternal, divine side. Below the Psychic Barrier, you experience the confines of limited earthly life—time and space.

Your lower mental-body contains your critical mind, reason, measurements, facts, comparisons, contrasts, judgment, blaming, dogma, ideology, beliefs, thoughts, ideas, intellectual intelligence, and interpretations. This is your monkey-mind. You develop it at school. Much of your operative earthly reality is created here.

Your empirical ego-self focalizes in your lower mental-body. Your earthly sense of self in society resides at the 3rd rung.

As you evolve, your mind matures to access your divine nature. Your upper mental-body develops. You begin to study conscience, integrity, discretion, discernment, morality, and character building. These basic trainings open you to consciously experience your Soul. With the development of your upper mind, you begin transcending earthly realms.

Your earthly mind makes a better servant than master. Your mind is a useful ally when you train it to access your divine levels.

The difficulty is that your mind is designed for earthly realms. It resists the foreign realms of your divine bodies. Transcending limited duality to infinite supply is against the mind's nature. Your rational, lower mind may at first see positive thinking and Truth-training as illogical, childish, artificial, or dishonest.

However, when you discipline your mind to positive thinking, you align with God. You then access infinite healing supply, spirit, and your God states.

Coming down the vibratory scale of your God Ladder to the 2nd rung, you discover your emotional body. It loosely correlates with your mid-abdomen chakra. Here the learning curriculum is feelings, healthy boundaries, entitlement, communication, issue identification, and conflict resolution skills.

Emotions are a bridge between your physical and mental levels. Emotions help you identify what you like and don't like; what you desire and disdain; what you want and fear; who you are and who your are not. At the 2nd rung, you process your personal history. Emotions help you digest the events of your life.

Descending further to the 1st rung of your God Ladder, your physical body contains your sensory experience: taste, touch, sight, hearing, and smell. Your 1st rung loosely correlates with your root chakra at the base of your spine. It houses your skills for survival and instinct.

Through your physical body, you experience the material world of duality: up/down, hot/cold, left/right, male/female, pleasure/pain, etc. Beauty, mobility, nurturing, and growth can come through your physical body.

At birth, when you receive your lower 3 bodies, you enter the realm of matter. It is a privilege for spirit to marry matter through the human experience. The richness and variety of earthly life are not available other places in the multiverse.

It is also a privilege for matter to marry spirit. Spirit elevates and ennobles matter, infusing it with conscious awareness. Spirit informs earthly matter of higher, divine realms.

Your lower 3 earthly levels are influenced by facts. By contrast, your upper 4 divine levels are directly connected to Truth. The origin of healing is your divine side.

Your divine bodies are anchored in the Real. The Real is unchanging, infinite, and eternal. Your earthly bodies are temporary and passing. Earthly reality is unreal—a transient, insubstantial dream. However, it must still be dealt with as long as you are in flesh.

In today's world, we are turned inside out and upside down— disoriented from our True Source. Mother never mentioned you have 7 elbows! The God Ladder helps you re-engage with your infinite healing Supply and your complete anatomy.

It may be disturbing to realize you have 7 elbows rather than just one—7 operational levels, 7 reality states, 7 identities. Certainly, it requires increased coordination to mobilize and integrate a system 7 times more complex.

However, your harvest of wisdom and healing exponentially multiplies as you claim dominion over your entire God Ladder. Your complete spiritual anatomy is your birthright.

One definition of healing is circulation. As your consciousness expands, it circulates among your 7 bodies. Your healing increases. Use your God Ladder to increase healing and expand awareness.

A key to happiness is feeling connected. Through your God Ladder, you connect with yourself, your God, your many powers, and your many worlds. As your dominion increases sevenfold, may your wisdom, joy, and healing multiply—at least sevenfold!

God Ladder Calisthenics

It's a question of cleaning then developing spiritual sense!
See
Beyond phenomena.
—Jelaluddin Rumi

All 7 levels of your God Ladder are active all the time. However, you may only be conscious of the level where your identity focuses in a particular moment.

In God Ladder calisthenics, you stretch your consciousness, moving your identity up and down your Ladder. You witness your life from all 7 levels: physical, emotional, mental, intuitional, Soul, personal God Self, and infinite God Source.

You name your experience from each of the 7 rungs of your God Ladder. The 7 stories of a single event may radically differ! Your emotions may tell one story; your mind another. Your body and spirit may tell additional stories!

Practice self-interviewing all 7 aspects of your complete anatomy to keep your God Ladder clear, open, and circulating healing energies.

God Source is the Big Kahuna. It contains your infinite supply of healing, intelligence, and resource. It is the part of you that is the miracle worker. It is your refuge and renewal. Your God Self and Soul connect you with your God Source.

Be alert throughout the day. Notice where you are on the God Ladder. Expand your awareness to include your divine bodies and increase your healing supply. God is just a thought away. Remember God.

Pain can trap you inside your earthly bodies. It can trick you into believing you are your limited earthly identity. Use your God Ladder to access all your powers.

Your God Source, with its infinite supply, intelligence, and healing, never leaves you. However, you may leave it if you forget your True Identity. Genesis 1: 27 says, "God created humankind in his own image." Remember who you are. Wherever you are, God is. Wake up and remember!

Repeat often, I am God. I am goodness. I am love divine. I am healing. I am wisdom. I am in all that is. Use your God Ladder to receive all the gifts of your complete anatomy!

FACTS VS. TRUTH

We look at life through the eyes of illusion. Then we make life
wrong for not meeting our expectations.
—Rabindranath Tagore

Continuously ask, What is Real? What is True?
Where is my power? Where is my Source?
—Judith Larkin Reno, Ph. D.

Where is Your Power?

What appears and disappears is not real.
—Sri Ramana Maharshi

This chapter continues your **Truth training** that began with Krishna's
Pearls of Wisdom. Principles of Truth are the foundation of your
healing. Your power always lies in Truth and God Source.

Practice discerning the difference between facts and Truth. Facts
exist inside the earthly realm. Truth originates in your divine bodies.
It opens your power-lines to God's infinite healing supply. Truth can
re-create your earthly facts.

When battling major illness, don't be distracted by the
overwhelming negativity of your situation. Stay connected to your
power. Truth connects you to God's healing, regardless of the negative
facts of your condition.

I can't enumerate how many times the "facts" said I was about to
die. Years later, I am alive and well. My story is one of millions. Miracles

abound. You can follow medical advice without giving your power to negative medical facts.

To find Truth, ask What's passing? What's permanent? The facts of your situation will pass. It's guaranteed. All things in life are temporary. By contrast, Truth is eternal.

The laws of Truth create and inform each of your seven bodies. The reverse is not true. For example, the lowest vibratory rung of your God Ladder, the physical, is not present at the level of Source— except as unmanifest essence and potential. By contrast, Truth is a powerful operative force at all seven levels of your complete anatomy.

You can reconstruct your earthly "facts" by applying principles of Truth to your earthly condition. You can change your experience of pain and disease.

Suffering exists in the earthly realm. There is no suffering in your divine realm. Bring divine Truth to your earthly facts and you can reduce your suffering.

Earthly facts change according to your perception. For example, wood appears solid to the casual observer. Solid material form is an earthly illusion—a basic assumption of earth-life that you rarely question.

However, to a quantum physicist, wood is a seething mass of atoms, jumping and moving chaotically. The same "solid" object appears fluid. If you change your viewpoint from Newtonian to quantum physics, the facts change.

Similarly, the "facts" of your life change if you view them from different rungs of your God Ladder. Regarding a single event, your body will not tell the same story as your emotions, mind, Soul, personal God Self, or impersonal God Source. Each rung provides a radically different reality. Use your God Ladder to change and refresh your view of earthly facts.

Quantum principles of observer participancy say that the viewer influences the facts—actually changing them. For example, when two people sequentially view the same apple, they see two different apples. In addition, there literally are two different apples! The apple itself changes depending upon the viewer.

Wayne Dyer says, "When you change the way you look at things, the things you look at change." If you bring high velocity, divine consciousness to your earthly facts, you can change them!

Facts also change according to the instrument of measurement. For example, light can be measured both as a particle and as a wave depending on the measuring device. Facts literally change when you use your Soul Vision and God Glasses!

Old standards of material science are crumbling as the new quantum paradigm emerges. Through Heisenberg's Uncertainty Principle, we now can prove that 2+2=4. Using the same principle, we can also prove that 2+2 ≠ 4!

Entering the realm of paradox, today science is facing the limits of the concrete mind and traditional scientific method. "Facts" are not what they used to be!

Live long enough and you will notice that facts change with time. One researcher says that you should exercise three times per week. Months later, another researcher reveals that you should exercise every day to be healthy.

"Facts" about healthy diet change continually. One year, "scientific facts" say you should eat an egg a day. The next year, cholesterol is discovered. Scientific research says you should eat two eggs per week.

Like the fragrance worn by a beautiful woman, facts are fleeting. The fragrance is enchanting and lingers in the room after the woman leaves. However, eventually it evaporates and is gone—like a dream.

If you anchor your foundation in the physical world, your house will evaporate. Earthly facts are insubstantial and transient. Clearly, they are not the source of your power.

The mundane world of facts can produce a hypnotic effect, holding you in a self-limiting trance. If society says miracles don't happen—and you agree in your hypnotic trance—you may remain pain-bound. If your tribe ignores the limitless potential of your divine nature, you may limit your own healing.

However, if you awaken from the trance, infinite healing is possible. Sacred tantra teacher Robert Frey says, "A miracle is not the suspension of natural law, but the operation of a higher law in love-based consciousness." It behooves you to make friends with the higher law!

Facts are the province of your monkey-mind. In the words of the famous Stash teabag, "What you know is more than what you think." Transcend your mind to find your limitless resource of healing Truth.

The mind cannot handle the paradoxes of the higher rungs of your God Ladder. Truth often contradicts facts. The higher rungs require faith and spiritual IQ.

You can mobilize positive change in your life if you invest in Truth while you work to improve negative facts. When you source from God, there is an answer to every problem—despite external appearances.

Truth has a different feeling from facts. The opposite of lack and limit, Truth is limitless abundant supply. Truth transports you to God. It returns your center, hope, and trust.

Truth is non-polarized, non-judgmental, detached, and unconditionally loving. It is always constructive and Self-affirming. You hear it in the "still, small voice" of your Soul.

On the 9/11 Investigation Commission, Richard Ben-Veniste said, "A fact is the point at which you agree to let the investigation stop." I'm calling for deeper investigation! I invite you to self-interview your entire God Ladder until you discover Truth.

Don't give your power to pain. Retrieve your power from external facts. Continuously ask, What is True? You will find your power there.

Truth Liberates You from Pain Jail

Don't let life hold you hostage.
—Judith Larkin Reno, Ph. D.

The enlightening task before us is to wake up to the realization that we are absolutely free; to consciously continually remember who we are.
—Sri Ramana Maharshi

Truth is your key out of pain jail. With Truth, the entire universe—its power, intelligence, and healing—all are yours. Remember the glories of your God Source.

There is no pain in your divine bodies. There is no polarity or resistance. The nature of Truth and your Divine Self is non-duality, harmony, love, and oneness. How can oneness fight against itself? How can we oppositionalize if there is only "us"?

By contrast, pain lives inside the earth's dualized world. Pain increases as resistance increases. Think of the toaster lighting up as electrical resistance increases in its coils. Pain can signal resistance to Truth somewhere in your God Ladder. A false-belief or negative emotion may be blocking healthy circulation.

Pain contracts your attention. Spirit expands it. If you fixate on pain, you become a spiritual amnesiac, forgetting your infinite God-nature. You can easily contract your identity into your pain.

Pain intensifies the more you identify with it. If you firmly anchor your identity in your Divine Self, your identity expands. Pain automatically diminishes.

Practice God Ladder calisthenics expanding your consciousness. Move up your God Ladder into Divine embrace. Surrender to God's will. You can honor the facts of your disease without allowing them to define you.

Monitor the source of your identity. Are you True Sourcing from God? Or, are you false-sourcing from pain and disease?

If you source from external events, you live in a shallow, unfulfilled, frustrating trap. The factual level of your life is not your True Source. Your True Source is God. Don't squander your energy on external reality. Invest instead in your God connection. Sri Ramana Maharshi says, "Turn your vision inward and the whole world will be full of supreme spirit."

To get out of pain jail, construct refuge in Truth. As the *Bible* says, "Truth will set you free."

Appearance vs. Reality

> *Life's but a walking shadow, a poor player*
> *That struts and frets his hour upon the stage,*
> *And then is heard no more.*
> —Shakespeare, *Macbeth*

Row, row, row your boat,
gently down the stream
Merrily, merrily, merrily.
Life is but a dream.
—Folk Song

Buddhists call earthly life the unreal, always-changing samsara. It is an illusion, an insubstantial dream—a passing puff of smoke. Life on earth is the "un-reality show."

Deal with mundane life. But don't confuse it with your identity or the Real.

The Real does not change. What comes and goes is not Real. Find the place inside you that is unmoved by all of life's hurly-burly—untouched by pain. Go there. Construct refuge in the quiet, still place inside. It is Real. The Real resides beyond life's distracting, temporal traffic.

Your physical body, emotions, thoughts, and facts exist in the illusory realm of earthly appearance. They are clouds passing over the sun. Let them pass over you like wind or weather. Don't confuse them with your True Identity.

Remember the beautiful Vedic prayer: "Lead me, Oh Lord, from darkness to Light, from the unreal to the Real, from chaos to Beauty, from death to Immortality."

When you affirm Truth, you are no longer at the effect of your life. You don't allow the facts of your disease to hold you hostage. You move beyond them. You move from pain to power, from victim to victor. You move from the unreal to the Real.

False Beliefs

Truth has no special time of its own. Its hour is now—
always.
—Albert Schweitzer

Fear blocks spirit.
—Aluna Joy Yaxk'in

The opposite of Truth, false beliefs are negative, lack-and-limit thinking. They create scarcity, ignorance, and suffering. They live in your lower mental-body, which is your critical monkey-mind. False beliefs are cognitive distortions that negatively color and twist your reality.

These earth-bound illusions are unexamined assumptions that you hold as true. Impeding a mature relationship with God, false beliefs can prevent happiness and healing. Some favorite false belief are "I'm not enough." "God forgot me." "I am cut off from infinite healing supply."

False beliefs can come from your family of origin, society, the media, institutions, church, school, friends, the collective, immaturity, or past lives. Deep, unconscious, false beliefs often either imitate your parents or oppositionalize from them. Either way, parents shape your unconscious beliefs.

In maturity, you individuate from your parents. You become conscious of false beliefs. Healing is becoming conscious.

Your healthy goal is to be awake in the dream, lucidly penetrating earth's fantasy. Sleepwalking through life is bondage to the past. If you are spiritually asleep, you suffer.

To awaken, use Krishna's Pearls of Wisdom. Reading the list aligns you with Truth. It restores your power.

You may notice resistance to certain Truths in Krishna's Pearls of Wisdom. Resistance identifies your false beliefs. Resistance signals where illusion is blocking the healing flow through your God Ladder.

The pain of your personal history and the facts of your earthly journey can hook you. Resolve the attached place and your pain diminishes. You can honor the facts of your life, without confusing them with the Truth of your identity.

You can witness your pain, without investing your belief in it. Instead, believe in the Truth of your infinite healing supply. Believe in God's wisdom.

Keep alert for **the following false beliefs** that take you away from Truth and jail you in pain. Immediately, reverse false beliefs into positive statements of Truth.

- **All-or-nothing thinking**. With black/white thinking, you see things at either end of the spectrum. There is no moderation or balance. With this rigid, extreme thinking, there is only one right way. Right/wrong polarization ensures failure, since life is not about perfection. Perfectionism is a mental disease. The healthy challenge is to find Buddha's Middle Road. Identify extremist logic when you hear it. "Always" or "never" sometimes flag this common mental distortion. Extremist thinking says, "The procedure failed, therefore I'm going to die." Remedy false thinking with positive thinking, "God's in charge. There must be a good reason for the delay. My healing is coming in God's way and in God's time."
- **Generalization**. With this false belief, you take a single negative experience and condemn your entire life or being. You assume a never-ending series of problems because of one problem. "Always" and "never" can also flag this cognitive distortion. False belief: "The procedure failed. I never have success." Transmute to "There must be another way to healing. With God's help I will find it." Notice when you think, "There's never enough." Return to Truth with, "Through God, I have infinite supply. All that I need is here, now."
- **Catastrophizing.** Here you exaggerate and magnify possible negative future events. You assume the worst catastrophe. Hyperbole is great for dramatic effect in story-telling. However, be careful you don't become a drama queen regarding your treatment. Assuming that you know the future is grandiose. Your future is in God's hands—not yours. Back off from catastrophic thinking. Surrender to your trust-worthy God.
- **Taking your life personally**. Shift your perspective when you assume that the gashes you suffer in life are personal. Take life seriously—but not personally. Difficulties come to every human. Avoid, "I did something wrong; therefore, I'm being punished with disease." Correct your false belief with, "I am a perfect child of a loving God. There are no accidents. I trust God's wisdom and plan for me."

- **Obsession.** Fixating on a single negative detail can be a form of toxic self-shaming. Notice when you excessively ruminate without resolution. Avoid the self-perpetration of obsession. Break the brain-lock. Expand your contracted focus to include divine realms. Trust your ultimate parent, God. Distract your mind with prayer and positive affirmation. Replace obsessive thoughts with gratitude for life's blessings. Read your Gratitude Lists. See the chapter on "Gratitude."

- **Self-discounting.** Be careful not to reject praise or compliments with false humility. If you do a good job, accept praise. You are God in human form. Allow your God Self to receive well-deserved praise through you. Let the praise-power feed and strengthen every level of your God Ladder.

- **Mind reading.** Don't assume you know what your partner, thinks, feels, or believes. If you have questions or doubts, ask him for answers. Gain clarity. Make no assumptions about other people. It's grandiose to assume you know when you don't.

- **Fortune-telling.** With this false belief, you predict that things will go wrong as a defense against trying. The false belief says, "Why bother trying. It's not going to work." The True belief says, "I don't know if it will work or not. However, I will follow wherever God leads me. I will give it my best try. I claim the highest and best results."

- **Futurizing.** Imagining a painful future event is the fast-track to fear and anxiety. Train yourself to stay in the present. Be here now. Let the future take care of itself. Most of our imagined fears are not what actually happens. Learn to place your future in God's hands. Surrender your cares.

- **Emotional reasoning.** This happens when you assume your negative emotions are facts. For example, "I feel inferior. That proves I'm inferior." With this false belief, you project your emotions onto the landscape of your entire life. Instead of using twisted emotional logic, unhook from negative emotions. Don't allow them to rule your life. Ride the dragon of detachment up your God Ladder. Take refuge in Divine Good. Consciously, call your life and yourself good.

- **Shoulding on yourself.** Should statements are a way of self-shaming. They lock you in the pain jail of perfectionism. Shoulding can perpetuate unrealistic expectations, misplaced idealism, and false spirituality. Shoulds can separate you from healthy reality, your instincts, and healthy desire. False giving is not healthy. Replace what you "should" do with what you truly want to do. You are God in human form. Trust your True desire. It comes from God.

- **Shouldering.** Are you taking too much responsibility for others, yourself, events, life, or things? This is a form of false-godding, setting yourself up as god. With this cognitive distortion, there is no room for a legitimate God connection. The underlying illusion can be a lack of trust. Perhaps you have not yet invented a trust-worthy God. Replace false responsibility with surrender to God's plan. Replace performance with trusting your honest desire. Allow yourself to be weak and tired. Rather than pushing and shouldering, rest. Love yourself the way you are—warts and all. Don't try so hard. Put your burdens down. Let God carry them. Know when to pick up responsibility and when to surrender it.

- **Labeling or name-calling.** This defense mechanism is a quick regression to childhood and childishness. It is a way to gain the illusion of power. It sacrifices legitimate self-authority. Practice seeing everyone as a perfect child of God, despite negative appearances. Everyone is always doing his best, regardless of the appearance. When you feel yourself oppositionalizing, keep a soft heart. See the other person with compassion for his pain or ignorance.

- **Blaming.** There is a difference between naming and blaming. Naming is detached, objective, egoless, clear perception. With blaming, there is moral judgment, attachment, and condemnation. Usually there is also inappropriate emotional discharge, targeting, or dumping. The negative energy attached to blaming is gummy, heavy, dark, and egotistical. It may convey victimhood. Replace blaming with compassion and transcension. Name and discern. Speak clearly of any injustice. Then take action to protect yourself and remedy the situation.

- **Judging.** There is a difference between judging and discerning. With discernment, you simply identify and tell the truth—whether positive or negative. Discernment is an objective qualitative assessment. It is naming without blaming. It comes from a clean perspective and the heart of compassion—characteristics of the Soul. It also comes from detachment, a quality of your God Self. By contrast, the energy of judgment—like blaming—is moralistic, gummy, heavy, egotistical, and negative. Judgmentalness conveys an attitude of rejection, separation, and "better than." Change judgmentalness to humility, e.g., "Who am I to judge you? That's God's job, not mine." Then, protect yourself against untrustworthy people and situations as best you can.

- **Spontaneous regression.** When your unresolved wounds from childhood trauma activate, you may spontaneously regress to childhood in an instant. If you self-interview, you will witness the conveyer belt moving you back in time. You will see yourself as tiny and powerless, like a child. Some spontaneous regressions actually take you back to unresolved trauma from a past life. Notice when you lose touch with the present. Automatic regressions can be very subtle. Notice when your voice gets tiny, your posture shrinks, or you feel unempowered. Return to your healthy entitlement. Know yourself as a perfect child of a loving God. Affirm your worthiness, legitimacy, and deservability. Some people regress to the temper tantrums of childhood. Keep alert for regressive, childish behavior and thoughts. Instead of childish eyes, see through your God Glasses and Soul Vision.

- **Dramatizing.** Notice when you use hyperbole and exaggeration. Your inner drama queen may be trying to compensate for a lack of healthy narcissistic supply. Do you need attention? Back off the urgency and drama. Give yourself extra love and acceptance. Ask your beloveds for extra love and support. Remember, you are not the first to experience pain. Disease, pain, and death are normal parts of human life.

- **False contracts.** Notice when you say yes and mean no. Are you trying to earn love through manipulation, codependency, false spirituality, and false giving? False giving is when you give from an empty cup. Your life won't work unless you establish it in integrity. Give to yourself first.

- **False-sourcing.** This cognitive distortion happens when you confuse your earth-bound life with your God Source. If you false-source from yourself, other people, or events, you will suffer endlessly. Instead, True-source from your internal, divine Source. With God, there is always infinite supply, healing, and wisdom.
- **False-godding.** Be careful not to turn your disease or pain into your god. Don't shut-down to the beauty in the room, the people who care for you, and God's plan for you.
- **Self-godding.** Be careful you don't false-god from yourself. It is grandiose to inappropriately rescue or enable others. Trust God's plan beyond your own. It is also self-godding to be too strong when you feel weak. Ask for help. Reach out. You are not alone.

Use these tips to retrieve your power from false beliefs. Bring the heart of compassion to yourself as you learn to care for your entire God Ladder.

Your power lies in your divine nature. Find your Truth. Continuously monitor internal scripts for positive and negative. Facts are often negative. Truth is always positive. Weed out negative, false beliefs. Affirm the Truth.

Listen to the facts of your medical situation. However, don't give your power to them. Invest in Truth.

Your God Glasses

> *It's amazing how the universe rearranges itself to fit your reality.*
> —Bumper Sticker

A student asked Sri Nisargadatta how he could believe in God when the world is full of disease and disaster. The great Indian sage replied, "In my world, nothing ever goes wrong." He knew the secret of wearing God Glasses!

Your God Glasses shift your perspective from earthly to divine. They transport you up your God Ladder. When you look through the eyes of eternity and infinity, your problems become small. Huge cataclysms instantly shrink.

Wearing God Glasses, you step into your Time/Space Machine. See your problem from 1,000 years in the future or from another planet. The shift in perspective unhooks you from your problem. Seen in the grand scheme of things, your problem becomes insignificant.

With God Glasses, everything looks positive. You see the larger plan. There is a reason for everything—to the tiniest detail of life.

You reframe from scarcity to abundance, from false belief to Truth. You know that God doesn't make mistakes. You trust God's plan beyond your own. Surrendering the narrow judgments of your ego-mind, you open to receive miracles.

When you're in the hospital or going through long-term illness, daily difficulties can exhaust you. To move, to see, to hear, and to communicate—basic elements of life—may become onerous or impossible. It's easy to lose positive thinking.

Negativity is an all-out alert that you have lost your way. Use your God Glasses to restore your God connection. Remember Einstein saying, "I want to think like God."

Wearing God Glasses, you are in the presence of holy wisdom. The world is meaningful and loving. There is no negativity or isolation. Everything makes sense. Fear and anxiety drop away. There is infinite supply.

God's universal, infinite perspective restores your sanity and hope. In *Anatomy of Hope: How People Prevail in the Face of Illness,* Dr. Jerome Groopman from Harvard Medical School cites research that positive belief and expectation release endorphins in the brain. Endorphins are natural painkillers. Wearing God Glasses can reduce your pain.

Dr. Deepak Chopra advocates improving your "internal biochemical pharmacy" by accessing God. In *Quantum Healing: Exploring the Frontiers of Mind/Body Medicine,* he presents medical studies proving the power of positive thought in healing.

Nurse and famous singer Naomi Judd used positive thinking to recover from catastrophic illness. She wore her God Glasses. She describes her miraculous journey to recovery in *Naomi's Breakthrough Guide.*

Neuro-science has proved that repeatedly focusing on positive thought actually reconstructs your brain! In *The Mind and the Brain,* psychiatrist Jeffrey Schwartz says regular one-pointed attention holds the brain's neural circuitry in place. Due to the brain's neuroplasticity, you redesign your brain when you see through your God Glasses.

Positive thinking improves your energy systems, your biochemistry, and your neural pathways! The moment you notice lack-and-limit thinking, negativity, or false beliefs, reach for your God Glasses. Affirm Truth, regardless of negative appearances.

If the negative thought is, "I have to go in the hospital again. This time, I'm afraid I'll die." Replace it with, "God has a perfect plan for me. I totally trust God and surrender to his will. Everyone gets to die. When it's my time, I will go with God's strength as my strength. I choose trust in God over fear."

Wear your God Glasses even while you sleep! Make them a permanent part of your spiritual wardrobe. The well-dressed spiritual anatomy need only wear God Glasses, a string of Krishna's pearls, and a smile!

Your Truth Compass

> *One definition of God is Perfection is everywhere—always.*
> —Judith Larkin Reno, Ph. D.

There are days when you can't find your God Glasses, divine perspective, or positive thinking. To realign with God Source, use your **Truth Compass**: *Perfection is everywhere—always.*

How does this one basic Truth apply to your painful situation? Keep turning the Rubik's cube of your "impossible" situation, until you discover the way in which it is perfect.

For example, if you break your arm, apply your Truth Compass: How is breaking your arm perfect? Perhaps a broken arm will slow you down, so you can "smell the roses." You may learn to enjoy your life. Slowing down might protect you, so you don't hurt yourself in a worse way. Perhaps, you will do some reading you wouldn't otherwise do. Or, you might meet a nurse who will change your life forever. Or vice versa! There are many possibilities.

Just as a ship uses a compass to stay on course, the Truth Compass keeps you aligned with God's infinite healing supply.

Negativity is the captain of illusion. Your job is to stay positive even in the face of apparent doom. This doesn't mean you can't be mad, sad, or frightened. It just means, you identify the negativity, name it, process it, resolve it, and sail on. Don't stay stuck in negativity.

Staying on course requires vigilance. Notice when victim, helplessness, hopelessness, orphan, worthlessness, discouragement, or depression appear. Use your Truth Compass to turn your thoughts to True Source.

Your Truth Compass helps you discern the following:

- Facts from Truth
- Appearance from Reality
- Your earthly self from your Divine Self
- False beliefs from Truth
- Lack-and-limit consciousness from infinite supply
- Negative thinking from positive thinking

Continuously reorient to the perfection of every moment, no matter how abysmal it may appear. A mangled physical body or a chaotic emotional condition may be factual. However, these facts need not own you.

In Truth, you are perfect. Though you may not understand it, your situation is perfect. Trust the Truth of your situation, not the facts. When you consciously anchor in Divine Self, your identity shifts. You access infinite healing supply.

When you align with God, anything is possible. The qualities of God—omnipresence, omniscience and omnipotence—are yours.

Follow your Truth Compass. Sail into the realm of limitless possibilities. Open your thinking to God. Allow an inrush of healing energy.

Healing Meditation

Let pain be a call to prayer.
—Judith Larkin Reno, Ph. D.

When you face a healing problem, gather the facts of your situation. See the facts clearly. Feel the pain. Notice the trapped, limited places.

Then, meditate. Ask God to heal you. See your situation through new eyes. Put your God Glasses on and see through the eyes of Truth. Return to the Real. Go up your God Ladder, dropping your earthly identities, one level at a time. Regenerate through your infinite God Supply.

Healing Meditation

Inhale. Exhale. Relax and smile. Release all tension in your physical body. Command the tightness to let go. Relax from the top of your head to the bottoms of your feet. Let go and let God support you. Release your physical body.

Inhale. Exhale. Relax and smile. Release your emotions—no matter how justified and compelling they may be. Just let them go. See them evaporate from your energy field. They rise like dark soot as they leave you. See a still pool of sparkling clear water remain.

Ascend your God Ladder. Enter your mental body. Hear the chaotic, noisy, mind chatter. Feel the buffeting winds of negativity, worry, judgment, and desire. Gently inhale. Exhale. Relax and smile. Drop your squirrelly, busy, tangled thoughts into the clear pool of stillness. See them dissolve. Relax your mind. Enjoy the quiet. It feels good to drop all your problems into the healing pool. Feel the hand of God soothe and smooth away all the cares of the day. Enter the calmness.

When you are ready, continue up your God Ladder until you reach your God Source. Enter the Great Chamber of God's Presence.

Imagine you are standing in the full glory of God. See God's effulgent Diamond Sparkle Divine White Light. God's power is almost more than you can bear. Melting in God's love, you drop into his embrace.

Feel your burdens lift off. Hear the cosmic sound of Truth whirl by you—resounding throughout the universe. It is like a tuning fork vibrating every particle and planet. Safe in God's love, you experience renewed power.

As you merge with God's great creative energy, you plug into infinite supply. In oneness with God, you feel his infinite intelligence, healing, and supply as your own.

Bring these divine energies down into your mental, emotional, and physical bodies. Feel all lack and limitation dissolve. See all barriers to your healing melt away.

Total healing is yours now. Glorious, healing energy flows down, flooding your mental, emotional, and physical bodies with Diamond-Sparkle Healing Light. Darkness evaporates in the healing Light.

See and feel your physical body as perfect. Infinite health circulates throughout your body, now. You are completely healed. Feel the lightness of your body. The heavy weights lift off. Every cell rejoices.

Aglow with healing radiance, you vibrate with renewed vitality. Dwell for a moment in your perfection.

Affirm the greatness of your being through God union. Gratefully accept your healing. Surrender your life into God's hands. As a perfect child of a loving God, you completely trust your God Supply.

With thanks and great love, you say goodbye to your God Chamber. Bring all the healing back with you, as you begin your return to earthly life. You are totally refreshed, renewed, and rebuilt as you re-enter your body—freshly consecrated.

Take a moment to dwell in your revitalization.

Your inner work, aligning with God presence, acts as a consciousness brace. It redirects your neural pathways, biochemistry, and energy systems to produce change in your mundane circumstance. Accessing God Source can re-create the facts of your life. Bathing in the stream of limitless healing, you cleanse. Your life renews, regenerates, and restores.

Throughout the day, when your identity wants to jail itself in pain, train yourself to return to your infinite, healing refuge. Ask to see the perfection. Use prayer, invocation, meditation, visualization, Krishna's Pearls of Wisdom, your God Ladder, your God Glasses, Soul Vision, and your Truth Compass to return to your Divine Self.

Climb your God Ladder and claim your healing, daily. Merge with infinite God Supply. Feel the healing energies in your body. Bring the renewal of body, emotions, mind, and spirit back to your daily life.

My dear friend Rev. Kimberly Marooney is the author of the beautiful *Angel Blessings Oracular Cards*. She was in an "impossible" circumstance one day. She called and we talked about it, identifying the Truth and the facts of her situation. She is a true spiritual warrior. I'll always remember her saying, "I'm not going to let the illusion win!" Aligning with Truth, she set herself free.

You can too—with Truth on your side.

REFRAME PAIN TO POWER

Happiness is a choice. Anyone can have a happy life—
even in the face of catastrophe. Events need not define you or
your state of mind. Take back your power!
—Judith Larkin Reno, Ph. D.

Reframing Negative to Positive

Most people are as happy as they make up their minds to be.
—Abraham Lincoln

Reframing is the process of translating a negative into a positive. Reframing transmutes loss to triumph, trial to treasure. You look beyond pain to find your gain. This chapter strengthens your **reframing skills** as you apply Truth principles to medical situations.

Reframing uses your God Glasses and Truth Compass. They connect you to divine levels of infinite healing and expanded perspective. In addition, their positive thinking opens your earthly equipment to receive healing.

In reframing, you start with a positive assumption that whatever happens is for the highest good. Whatever happens, you call it good. Immediately, you shift from victim into victory.

Richard Bach says, "The mark of your ignorance is the depth of your belief in injustice and tragedy. What the butterfly calls the end of the world, the master calls a butterfly." That's reframing!

Here's another good reframe: When your hair is falling out due to chemo, instead of fixating on the loss, find the power. Say, "Isn't this wonderful! The fact that my hair is falling out proves that the medicine is working! The medicine wouldn't be killing my hair unless it was also killing the disease!"

To reframe, turn the negative situation in your mind until you discover its positive function. How is the negative experience serving you? What good can possibly come from this experiences? What are you learning through the pain? Once you see pain's gift, you feel empowered.

Reframing is power retrieval. You take back your power from pain. The more power you retrieve, the more energy you have for healing.

Reframing is treasure hunting. Hunting for the perfection, you affirm divine order rather than chaos. You turn loss into treasure, grief into a gift, the wound into wisdom.

To reframe from pain to power, throughout the day continuously **ask the following key questions**:

- Who am I? Am I my pain or Infinite Supply?
- Where is my power? In the pain? Or in my God Source?
- Where is God in this situation? Am I True Sourcing from God or false-sourcing from physical events?
- What are the facts? What is True? Am I anchored in Truth regardless of negative facts?
- How is this situation perfect?
- What am I learning?

A good reframe converts enemies to allies. For example, rather than focus on the pain of needles and medical procedures, see them as allies helping you to heal.

Let's say an infection delays a major medical procedure. Rather than dwell on your disappointment with the postponement, reframe. Marvel at how protected you are to detect the infection before it complicates your medical procedure!

A good reframe is no small skill. Finding the silver lining in the dark cloud requires spiritual intelligence. Buddha reframed so quickly and effectively that a violet instantly blossomed in place of the negativity!

Reframing Skills

Nothing is good or bad, but thinking makes it so.
—Unknown

When you frame a house, you construct the skeleton that will support the entire building. The complete house emerges from its frame. Similarly, when you frame the house of your consciousness, you lay the groundwork for your entire life. Your life emerges from your foundation principles.

If you start from positive assumptions that the universe is friendly and God is on your side, your life will be happy—regardless of circumstance. Assuming the positive, you find the gift of learning in every negative situation.

In reframing, you consciously construct a positive view of each negative experience. You see each negative situation as an opportunity for growth—a gateway to God. You flip the negative experience to find its positive benefits and opportunities.

To reframe, turn the puzzle pieces of your negative situation until you discover what you are learning. Suddenly, the picture turns positive. You see the perfection. You have an "aha" experience, followed by relief.

To strengthen your **reframing skills**, practice the following **3 rules**:

1. **Take responsibility for your life**. As Joan Rivers says, "Grow up!" From the level of the Soul Contract, there are no victims.
2. **Use your Truth Compass**. Ask how your painful situation reflects *Perfection is everywhere—always*. Keep turning the situation in your mind until you find the way it is perfect.
3. **Find the gift** in the pain. What are you learning through the pain? What is the gain beyond the pain?

In the 1st rule, being responsible for your life is not the same as blaming yourself or feeling guilty for negative events. The appearance level polarizes into right/wrong, good/bad moral judgment. At the level of Truth, we don't make mistakes. We simply have learning experiences.

You chose your life to the tiniest detail when you agreed to your Soul Contract prior to birth. Your Soul is wise and does not betray you. If your Soul gave you a challenge in this life, it is because you are strong enough to handle it.

You can choose to be responsible for your life or you can be a victim. Even if you don't believe in your Soul, from a practical level, choosing to be responsible for your life saves pain. Opposing divine law is a useless proposition. If you align with divine law, it will serve you—rather than exhaust you.

Being responsible is spiritual adulthood. The difference between an adult and a child is that the adult knows the limits. The adult respects the law. The adult knows how to grieve the limits and "Get over it," as Ms. Rivers would say.

In spiritual maturity, you accept life's limits. You live according to divine law. The moment you take adult responsibility for your life, you open to receive the wisdom gift inside the pain. Spiritual teacher Eckhart Tolle says, "True freedom and the end of suffering is living in such a way as if you had completely chosen whatever you feel or experience at this moment."

The 2nd rule of reframing is to use your Truth Compass to find the perfection. In what way is your painful experience perfect? What false beliefs and negativity must you drop to see the perfection? What are the benefits of the pain? What are the learning metaphors and symbols of your pain?

For example, imagine you are going for open-heart surgery. In what way is by-pass surgery perfect? A kaleidoscope of possible answers arises. Perhaps you are reassessing major issues of the heart, learning how to love. Maybe you are learning to be vulnerable and to receive love.

Perhaps you have triumphed over a lifetime of love illusions modeled by your parents and society. By trial and error, you've sorted through the illusions, until you have finally found true love. Now, you need a new heart to match your true beliefs. Or, perhaps you are learning to take heart and find courage in a new way.

When you know *Perfection is everywhere—always,* you realize that you are the perfect child of a loving God. In fact, you are God's favorite child! Your nature is to be lucky. To reframe pain to power, start with these assumptions.

Practice feeling lucky. When the illusion of unluckiness appears, affirm the perfection, here, now. Cultivate feeling blessed.

For example, in *Fiddler on the Roof,* another dinner guest surprises the impoverished Russian peasant wife at the family's already meager meal. She shakes her head. Looking heavenward—moving beyond facts—she affirms Truth. She insists, "Another blessing!"

What fine reframing! No matter what happens, affirm the perfection.

Tuesdays with Morrie by Mitch Albom gives a wonderful example of the 3rd rule of reframing—find the gift in the pain. Morrie is a terminally ill professor who shares his experience with his student during weekly visits. As Morrie's health declines, he becomes too weak to get out of bed. His student asks how Morrie endures the indignities of not being able to get to the bathroom.

Morrie replies, "It's comforting to have someone wipe your butt. It's like being an infant again when Mom cleaned the baby with powders and oils and extra love." Morrie reframes negative experience to positive. Rather than fight the inevitable, he enjoys it. He finds the gift. You can learn to reframe—because it feels better.

Keep speaking Truth and you will find the gift in the pain. Nothing can endure the Light of Truth, except Truth.

As you develop your reframing skills, transmuting negative to positive, you become like an elegant ballerina who turns on a point, instantly flowing in a new direction. Through selfless surrender to "what is," you align to serve God's will. You find freedom.

To reframe from negative to positive, simply ask, how do I want to see this event? Do I want to see it as negative, which turns me into a victim? Or, do I want to see it as a learning treasure, which creates me as a victor!

Perfection Is Everywhere—Always

See pain as a valuable teacher.
Accept your life as it is.
Take responsibility for events—
even if your agreement was made
in your Soul Contract
before you were born.
Find the perfection that's here, now.
Go deep.
Don't stop asking
until you find the gift in the pain.

Watching a Master Reframe

My imperfections and failures are as much a blessing from God
as my successes and my talents. I lay both at his feet.
—Mahatma Gandhi

Posters, bumper stickers, postcards, and office reminders that say "Breathe" owe their origin to Leonard Orr, the founder of Rebirthing. Leonard is a unique, germinal thinker. During the 1970's, he was the first Westerner to popularize "breathing." Amazingly, prior to that time, Americans were generally unconscious of breathing!

"Breathe" is an obvious—though evasive—wise expression. It has become deeply woven into our everyday culture. I remember Judge Ito preserving order in O. J. Simpson's murder trial by telling everyone to "Breathe."

When he toured the United States to teach Rebirthing, Leonard sometimes visited me. It was fun and often profound to be around him. He opened doors of fresh insight for me.

I remember one visit when, through a series of mishaps, it appeared that Leonard's life was falling apart. I felt panic and worry for my friend. Expressing my concern for the apparent upheaval, I imagined how depressed I would feel in the same situation.

However, Leonard wasn't worried at all. He was almost salivating when he replied, "Now the fun begins!"

I realized I was watching a master reframe. He knew that chaos brings new order.

Shadow Interview

> *Error is just as important a condition of life's progress as truth.*
> —Carl Jung

Your shadow is an unconscious, disowned element of your consciousness that may at first appear ugly. Shadow can present as anger, fear, sadness, grief, misfortune, pain, or disease.

In spiritual treasure hunting, you dive deep to find shadow's gift. Probing beneath surface events, you see shadow turn to Light. Behind the shadow, you encounter the hand of God. Pain is merely a teacher hired by your Soul to deliver a wisdom gift.

Jungian psychologists who specialize in integration are famous for saying, "The shadow knows. The shadow holds the gold."

For example, physical pain can uncover your identity confusion. Pain can liberate you from your mind/body trance, returning you to your God nature.

You must be alert to find the wisdom gifts of pain. Pain can occur in relation to any one of your seven bodies: physical, emotional, mental, intuitional, Soul, personal God Self, or impersonal God Source.

The trick to shadow work is to get in and get out quickly. Don't make shadow interviews a life-style. Rather, get the shadow's information for your self-knowledge. Then, move into changing in your life.

In shadow work, you learn through opposites. Shadow shows where there is no Light. Suffering delineates where you are trapped in illusion and false belief. Resistance signals what doesn't work. If you name the pain and identify your resistance, that information guides you to its opposite. Flipping false belief, you discover Truth.

The information from your shadow helps you make a course correction in thinking, emoting, and behaving. To **find the wisdom gifts of shadow pain, ask the following questions**.

Shadow Interview Questions

- What is the pain teaching me?
- What strength do I gain through this negative experience?
- What am I resolving through this pain?
- What are the benefits of being sick, mad, sad, or afraid?
- What do I avoid by being sick?
- If I weren't sick, what would I be doing?
- What people do I avoid by being sick?
- What people do I punish with my illness?
- What parent figure do I imitate, confront, oppose, or resolve through my pain?
- How is pain liberating me?
- How is it changing me?
- How is pain changing my values?
- How are my beliefs and basic life assumptions changing?
- What judgments am I dropping?
- How does pain change my identity?
- How is my relationship with God changing?
- How am I growing as a result of the negative experience?
- What false beliefs must I drop to see the perfection?
- What is the highest outcome for this experience?

Use your shadow to find the gold. Reframe shadow to Light, pain to gain. Treasure hunting for shadow gold and wisdom gifts, I often think of the Greek playwright, Aeschylus. He said, "In our sleep, pain that cannot forget falls drop by drop upon the heart. And in our despair, against our will, comes wisdom through the awful grace of God."

Gifts of Negative Emotions

Knowledge is structured in consciousness.
—Rig Veda

Emotional pain often accompanies physical pain. Find the gift of learning in each negative emotion. By claiming the wisdom gift, you transmute the pain to power.

Healthy anger's gift signals a boundary infraction. Anger shows when someone takes something that is yours or compromises your integrity. Through healthy anger, you affirm what is yours. You fight for justice. Anger helps you repel negative invasion.

Anger defines healthy boundaries and entitlement. It reveals the limits. Anger guarantees that you don't enmesh with or wall-off from others—including God. To maintain healthy boundaries, you must retrieve your power of "No"—a valuable gift of spirit.

For example, when you're furious at the limitations of disease or pain, separate your identity from the disease. Say "No!" to the disease/pain. Insist that disease/pain is not who you are. Know that you are entitled to something better. You are not a disease label. Your True Identity is in God, not in pain.

Healthy anger demonstrates your vital force. It focuses your strength to fight for survival or to defend justice.

The healthy function of sadness is to signal loss. Grief creates space for new life and new identity. Healthy sadness says goodbye to the past and opens the door to a new future. Grief provides the labor pains to birth your new identity.

To successfully negotiate loss, you must love God more than what you have lost. Through loss, you surrender to God's will. Sacrifice is sacramental. It consecrates your life. Through loss, you ride deeper into God's embrace.

To resolve grief, you must transcend events, trusting the Unknown—The Great Mystery. Transcending events is an irrational act. There is no motivation except God union and resolution of pain. You experience pain until you accept God's plan.

Enlightenment is a grief experience. The *Bible* says, "The price of wisdom is grief." Enlightenment is the loss of one illusion after another. You grieve each illusion to create space for new life and expanded identity. The ability to grieve defines spiritual adulthood.

Healthy fear tells you to proceed with caution. Fear shows a need for clarity, help, or information. Who or what is safe? What is right action? Where is my power?

Fear can teach faith. You overcome disproportionate, unhealthy fear by trusting in your Higher Power. Are you false-godding from disease labels and external events? You can have either your fear or faith.

The Anonymous Work says, "Resentment is the darkroom where you develop negatives." The healthy function of resentment is to signal a need for grieving, forgiveness, compassion (both for yourself and the offender), detachment, surrender, transcension, and God union. Followed to completion, the resentment cycle drives you back into the arms of God. It ensures your God union.

The wisdom treasure in healthy shame is humility. Humility sets healthy limits. Healthy shame helps you avoid the grandiosity of false-godding from yourself or others. You stop self-will run riot. Accepting life as it is—with all its flaws and limits—you surrender your addiction to perfection.

Healthy shame teaches the difference between your earthly will and God's will. As you surrender to God's will, you respect earthly limits.

What do you learn through self-pity? Self-pity is lost objectivity. Your identity collapses into sentimentalized personal drama at the expense of detachment. Self-pity is ultra self-conscious and self-absorbed.

Sniveling in narcissistic self-pity consumes your attention. The drama is so great that there is no room for God. You set yourself up as a false god. Moses said, "Mine is a jealous God." God won't tolerate a shared throne.

By setting yourself on the throne that belongs to God, you may be trying to receive the healthy narcissistic supply that is every infant's birthright. You may be compensating for a lack of healthy parental attention in your childhood. Excessive, repeated self-pity may indicate unresolved parental-abandonment issues.

If your parents weren't psychologically healthy, they didn't have enough emotional supply to give a baby. They didn't even have enough to give themselves. Without healthy narcissistic supply, the child experiences abandonment.

Becoming an adult is learning to self-nurture. Skills of appropriate self-adoration and self-parenting can replace the childhood deficit. In spiritual maturity, you create your own healthy internal mother/father archetypes. You stop waiting for a fantasy rescue.

Self-pity may be an emergency signal that you have lost your ultimate parent, God. To restore God alignment, when you feel self-pity, ask the following question: Who is my True Parent? Do I trust God's plan for me?

Each time you encounter a negative emotion that seems to be ruling your life, work with it until you find the gift of learning you are trying to give yourself. Practice treasure hunting. Look for the wisdom gifts. Behind the shadow, you will find gold.

Wisdom Gifts of Your Illness

> *The gift of physical pain is transcension. Pain forces you out of your physical identity into God union.*
> —Judith Larkin Reno, Ph. D.

> *Take wisdom from the wound.*
> —Judith Larkin Reno, Ph. D.

Spiritual friends of mine know that challenge is an opportunity to grow. They frequently ask, "What have you learned from your healing journey?" It is a fruitful question that I now ask you.

Feel free to borrow from my answers as you write your own in the space provided below. Remember to ask the question and renew your answers periodically in your healing journey.

What Have I Learned on My Healing Journey?

- To receive and to value love.
- To connect with God's infinite power, healing, and love.
- To construct God union as my refuge.
- To surrender to God's will, even though I don't understand it.
- To value God as the center of my life.
- To honor the limits of life—especially the boundary between life and death.
- To take my life seriously, but not personally.
- Not to confuse my identity with my life, pain, or disease.

- To be fully present on earth, but not to source from there.
- To appreciate the power of prayer in healing and saving lives.
- To disconnect from fear and concentrate on God when pain is great.
- To continuously ask, where is my power?
- To value the nature spirits who press their noses against the window at twilight to see how I'm doing.
- To treasure friendships in both the inner and outer worlds.
- To become guardian of my memories—protecting precious memories and releasing negative ones.
- To be thankful for the love affairs in life, even the ones that didn't work out. Those beloveds are frozen in time. We'll always be young and healthy in my memory. I can still access the joy and harvest the love we shared. The pain goes away. The love is forever.
- To value my body as God's interface with life. Without a human body, you can't feel the hug of a baby, hear the sound of Mozart, or experience a rose petal touching your cheek.
- To overcome cultural prejudice that sees death as defeat. Instead, I see death as graduation.
- I've learned all of life is God's grace.

Pain is a great teacher and giver of gifts. In spiritual treasure hunting, you penetrate the illusion of facts. Using Truth to reframe, you find the wisdom in your wound.

Collect the wisdom gifts of your healing journey. They are your spiritual gold. What has the healing journey taught you? **List the wisdom gifts from your healing journey below.**

_____

_____

_____

_____

_____

PAIN VS. SUFFERING

All earthly life is a light show—insubstantial and evanescent.
Don't confuse the light show with your identity.
—Judith Larkin Reno, Ph. D.

Let pain bring due reward of Light and Love.
Let the Soul control the outer form,
And life and all events.
—Alice Bailey, "The Mantra of Unification"

Suffering is Attachment to Pain

Attachment creates suffering. Attachment creates identity
confusion. Suffering is identity confusion.
—Judith Larkin Reno, Ph. D.

Pain is a natural product of life. It comes with your birth certificate. Pain is misaligned energy in your God Ladder signaling, "It's time to change." "Get help!" "Return to wholeness." Pain is part of earth's duality. As long as you are in flesh, you are subject to pain. It is unavoidable.

However, how much you suffer from pain is a matter of personal choice. Buddha draws an important distinction between pain and suffering. He says, when you attach to your pain, you create suffering.

Suffering increases when you attach your identity, self-worth, value, meaning, or ego to pain. Attachment to pain blocks the flow in your God Ladder—big-time.

You may not be able to control the pain in your life. However, you can control your suffering. Reduce your suffering by noticing your attachment to your pain. Consciously, disconnect and return to your True Source. Focus on God.

When pain is a devouring tiger, simply remembering God helps part of you to disconnect. Any freedom you create increases your God-link and decreases your suffering.

The healthy experience of pain is egoless and unattached. The pain moves through you without excessive emotions, stories, or judgment. D. H. Lawrence says,

> A small bird will drop frozen dead from a bough
> without ever having felt sorry for itself.

Animals process pain impersonally. The animal is an empty conduit through which pain passes without snagging on self-conscious scripts. Animals don't confuse their identity with the pain. They are automatically in the egoless, divine-witness state.

The distinction between pain and suffering is important.

- **Suffering is identity confusion.** When you fixate on pain, your identity fuses with it. You con-fuse your identity with your pain. You become the pain. Forgetting your True Identity, your suffering increases with your attachment to pain.
- **Suffering is separation from God**. Attachment to pain breaks your God connection. When you false-source from pain, you disconnect from True Source.
- **Suffering is ignorance.** Ignoring your divine side as refuge intensifies suffering. If you attach to pain, you forget the part of you that is untouched by pain. Absorbed in earthly identity, you ignore your Divine Source.

Monitor whether you are in pain or suffering. Attachment is the key. Pain is impersonal, like weather or electricity. When you take pain personally, you attach to it and increase your suffering.

Suffering often has emotional drama around it. In addition to the pain, you hear an exaggeratedly sad story in your head. Popular ego-scripts involve self-pity, helplessness, hopelessness, and victimhood. Resolve these scripts to ensure non-attachment to pain.

Judgment and blame are also indicators that you are in suffering rather than pain. They signal false beliefs and attachment. Suffering's mental and emotional overlays amplify physical pain.

To diminish suffering, let pain flow through you unobstructed, the way animals do—impersonally, without self-pity or judgment. Watch the pain move through you like water flowing downstream.

Practice witnessing your pain from a detached viewpoint. Witnessing puts a little distance between you and the pain, ensuring non-attachment.

In bi-level living, part of you stands outside your life watching, while the other part lives through events. You honor both your earthly and divine identities. Anchored in your divine witness, you see the pain through your God Glasses.

When Guruji was afflicted with pancreatic cancer, I asked if he were in pain. He answered, "The body will do what it does. It's not my concern. I must go on." He was unattached. He had a clear surrender to God's will. At the same time, he fought to live.

Self-monitor your attachment to pain. Don't allow it to consume you. You may not be able to change your pain. However, you can reduce your suffering.

Put a little distance between yourself and the pain. Put space around your pain. Practice non-attachment to your pain.

Preference vs. Attachment

I don't belong to myself.
—Buckminster Fuller

The difference between pain and suffering is attachment. Ego attachment turns pain into suffering. The ego-script "I want it my way" is very different from the God-centered script "I desire this and

I surrender to God's will." Attachment fractures your God-link, cutting you off from Infinite Supply.

Rather than attachment, cultivate preferences. Preferences are objective, unemotional, detached choices. With a preference, you witness your choice from divine perspective.

Preferences don't confuse your desire with your identity or your value. Using preference, you serve your desire without undue attachment to outcomes. You can accept either yes or no.

For example, imagine that you want candy. Using preference, if you don't get candy, you're still OK. Emotional sobriety and equanimity are qualities of non-attachment.

By contrast, if you are attached to your desire for candy, your world falls apart if you don't get it. You willfully *must have* candy. The candy owns you. False-sourcing from candy, it becomes your momentary god. You false-god from candy!

The energy of attachment is heavy, gummy, and excessive—even urgent and driven. If you want something too much, it is probably an attachment rather than true desire.

Attachments contract your energy field. Preferences expand your field to include God. Attachment can signal an addiction: physical, emotional, mental, or spiritual.

Saying "No. I don't want candy" is not negativity. Negativity conveys inappropriate emotional charge, judgmentalness, and ego. Negativity clogs and distorts your energy system, creating pain. Negativity disconnects your God Ladder.

Because you don't like chicken doesn't mean you are thinking negatively. However, be careful you aren't attached to your dislike of chicken. Don't hate the chicken. Don't give your power to the chicken! Attachment to your desire creates negative energy.

You may make selections on a menu. However, don't judge others who disagree with your choices. For example, don't make others wrong if they choose chicken rather than a vegetarian meal. Judgmentalness is a form of ego attachment.

Don't confuse your identity with your likes, dislikes, pain, or pleasure. Maintain a clear witness point as you make choices. Keep a little distance between yourself and your choices. Use your Soul-witness throughout the day to ensure non-attachment.

Keep in mind, if you allow your identity to become attached to your choice—technically speaking—you risk becoming a chicken in your next life!

Suffering Is Ignorance

Human misery is caused by ignorance of ourselves.
—Carl Sagan, Astronomer

When you are suffering ask, "What am I ignoring?"

Am I attached to my ideas of right and wrong, ignoring God's plan for me? Am I ignoring my infinite healing God Supply? Am I ignoring that ultimately nothing can harm me—not even death—because I am an immortal being? Am I ignoring that I belong here—for as long as I am here?

Self-interview each of the 7 rungs of your God Ladder to discover what you may be ignoring, including your physical, emotional, mental, intuitional, Soul, personal God Self, and impersonal God Source.

If you judge your pain, you ignore God's wisdom in giving you the pain. Common judgmental mind-scripts say, "This pain is bad." "I failed when I got sick." "God doesn't love me." The more judgment you have against pain, the tighter you bind to it. The more judgment you have, the more you suffer.

Pain exists for a reason. The reason may be universal, societal, familial, or personal. The reason may extend back thousands of lifetimes or into the future beyond human view. There are no accidents. Everything is connected. Everything is ordained by God.

Your mind may not see all the reasons for pain. Only your spirit can grasp God's plan for you.

God is a powerful partner in your healing. Don't ignore your God. Invite God to be your partner. Let God carry the pain load. It's arrogant to think you can carry all of it.

You suffer when you ignore your partnership with God. With God, all things are possible. The continuous movement between your earthly and divine sides—ignoring neither—creates health.

Ellen's Story

Happiness is an inside job.
—Judith Larkin Reno, Ph. D.

It helps to have models of healthy pain management—aside from birds and animals! God gave me Ellen. She demonstrated how to live a happy life while in terminal illness.

Ellen was diagnosed with cystic fibrosis as a child when the life expectancy was seventeen years old. She lived to be forty-six years old.

She lived an energetic, full life as an elementary school teacher. Ellen had a wonderful husband, children, supportive family, and great friends. She packed more into one lifetime than most people experience in several.

Ellen founded a summer camp for kids with cystic fibrosis. Having lived with a death sentence all her life, she wanted the kids to see living proof that statistics are just numbers. If she could beat the odds, so could they. She made medical history and invited others to follow.

Ellen led a CF support group, with an active web site. She received hundreds of e-mails weekly thanking her for being an inspiration.

I met Ellen a few years before her death. She was continually in and out of the hospital. Yet, when I saw her at social occasions, she looked vibrant. Her smile lit up the room. You would never guess the health difficulties she endured.

Despite her grueling health condition, she always had time for special surprises. After one of our Gateway gatherings, she made a fabulous photo album of the event as a gift for me. Typical of Ellen's involvement in life, she had taken a course on photo album design. The layout of the photo album was professional quality.

Ellen's ability to live in the present blew me away. How could she stand the pressure of never knowing when she'd land back in the hospital?

Ellen had a healthy ability to compartmentalize her life. She knew the value of celebration—and of living each moment. She didn't allow disease to rob her of daily delights. Her strong, clear focus was on enjoying each moment. When the hard times came, she dealt with them—not giving them any more attention than necessary.

Despite all Ellen endured, she never floundered in self-pity. She was busy appreciating her life, not complaining about it. I marveled at her positive attitude in the midst of challenges.

When the end came, Ellen faced it with characteristic courage. At her memorial service, her doctor's testimonial was moving. She had never seen anyone deal with pain with such equanimity as Ellen demonstrated.

While there was a sense of loss at Ellen's funeral, there was a greater sense of victory. Everyone who knew Ellen participated in it, like a triumphant conspiracy. "Job well done!" was the unspoken, internal chant. It was the feeling I get at a marathon, when the runners run a good race. Ellen was a spiritual athlete. She had defied the odds and won.

Curious about Ellen's resilience, I asked her father, "How did Ellen avoid self-pity? How did she keep her balance? How did she deal with pain so gracefully?"

Her father replied, "When Ellen was a little girl, she realized that she could lose her life at any time. She made a decision then to make every minute count. Life was too precious. She couldn't afford to waste it on self-pity. Her happiness was a conscious decision."

Ellen taught me that pain need not rob you of happiness.

GRATITUDE

*Stop whining about what you've lost. Get busy being thankful
that you had it!*
—Judith Larkin Reno, Ph. D.

Obsess on Your Treasure

There are a hundred ways to kneel and kiss the ground.
—Jelaluddin Rumi, Sufi Master

When I first got sick, I was clinging to life. Doctors thought I might have days or weeks to live.

I lived in the "Flat World," unable to sit up or get out of bed. My left arm was unusable due to pain. Because of tremors, pain, and too little strength in my right arm, I couldn't use the phone for five months. I was disconnected from friends and family. Even if I could have held the phone, I had no voice due to severe laryngitis.

My world had shrunk. I didn't have the energy to read or to watch television. Until then, I hadn't realized it took strength to watch TV!

For many months, I experienced "hell pains" and profound exhaustion. It was clear that I had to fight if I wanted to live. One night, my daughter Sara and I were discussing my challenges. There was no pleasure in my life. It was all pain.

She said, "You have to fight against the pain, Mom. Grab the tiniest sliver of pleasure in your life. Make it huge. Make it your entire world. Maybe all you have is the next inhale. Make it delicious! Pick a favorite color in the room. Make it your new best friend. Praise it. Adore it.

"Exaggerate each gift of beauty in the day—a beam of sunlight, a friendly smile, a cheery greeting card. Magnify every act of kindness by nurses or friends. Run each happiness through your memory repeatedly throughout the day.

"Grab the tiniest crumb of pleasure, like a starving man wrenches food from the throat of life. Your life depends on this, Mom. Claim your treasures, regardless of how puny they appear. Praise them lavishly. Express gratitude to them.

"With each treasure, become a proud explorer taking a new frontier. Plant a flag. Send out cheers. Hear the trumpet fanfare. Show your conquest to an admiring crowd.

"Claim your treasures, Mom. And, they will bring their friends. Slowly, gradually, your world will get bigger."

I took Sara's advice to heart. I'm glad I did. She was right!

Gratitude for Medical Care

I'm so paranoid, I always think people are trying to help me.
—Richard Allen, Comedian

Sometimes, I think the only prayer is "Thank you, God." I give thanks all day.

When I visit the clinic or doctor, rather than dreading the experience, I consider it God's grace. I enter with gratitude. No detail is too small for me to appreciate. I stay with gratitude—expanding it until bliss and serenity come.

I give thanks for my well-educated, first class doctor. She and her family suffered and disciplined so she could be here to help me. I am grateful for her skill and knowledge.

I am thankful for my nurses. Nurses are agents of God. They are God's hands in action.

Doctors and nurses work closely with angels, following God's guidance. They are nurturing and noble, wishing only to heal the patient and bring wellness. I give thanks to American medicine—some of the best in the world.

It's too easy to see treatment as the enemy. I could easily resent yet another medical procedure. Instead, I concentrate to keep clear of negativity. I focus on my gratitude.

At the clinic, I say, "I am happy to be here!" I give thanks for the strength that allows me to receive treatment. This loving medical care brings me one step closer to my goal of healing.

Medical care is a gift.

Your Daily Harvest Necklace

Acceptance and gratitude turn what we have into even more.
—Melody Beattie

Gratitude is healing. It is the express elevator straight to God's heart. You cannot overdo gratitude. William Blake said, "Gratitude is heaven itself."

Every day, I collect at least three blessings. They are like charms for a bracelet. I place them on my Daily Harvest Necklace to review each night as I fall asleep.

Be predatory searching for delights to fill your Daily Harvest Necklace. Pounce on anything that gives you the slightest joy, including a phone call, a note from a friend, the soft wind on your cheek, a TV show, birdsong, or the taste of food. The treasure may involve people. Other times, it may be an aesthetic experience, a valued emotion, or a happy memory.

My Daily Harvest Necklace adds adventure to my day. Throughout the day, I keep alert for pleasures. I assess and evaluate each event to see if it qualifies for my necklace. Collecting treasures is my pleasure secret.

As I sniff out blessings in my daily prowl, I continually look for the good things in life. Like a detective tracking a suspect, the necklace keeps me stalking joy all day. My Daily Harvest Necklace helps me "stop and smell the roses."

Even if I am bed-ridden, hospitalized, or immobilized, I can create my Daily Harvest Necklace. There's always a kindness from a nurse or a sweet gesture from the hospital staff that I can collect. I focus on the good things I have, not on what I don't have. The treasure hunt empowers me.

For each treasured memory, I place a living icon on my Daily Harvest Necklace. The image is alive with color and motion. Sometimes, the icon represents a whole scene, as if in a movie.

I always collect at least three icons for my Daily Harvest Necklace. Some days, there are a dozen treasures by bedtime. I look at my collection as it grows throughout the day.

At night, I wear my Daily Harvest Necklace to bed. It's fun to review each icon at the end of the day. The necklace glows in the dark. I fall asleep with the golden glow of the day's blessings around my head.

Below, list three treasures from today for your Daily Harvest Necklace:

_____

_____

_____

Your Gratitude Inventory

> *You fill up my senses, like a walk in the forest.*
> —John Denver, "Annie's Song"

Your Daily Harvest Necklace contains gratitude for specific gifts of the day. Your Gratitude Inventory includes a larger time scope. In it, you give thanks for the general blessings of your life.

In my Gratitude Inventory, I repeatedly include the following: my husband; children and their spouses; my family of origin; my healers and teachers; friends; my nation; civilization; my questing spirit; my relationship with God, Inner Guides, and angels; my beautiful body and its functioning parts. This part of the list changes from week to week!

I repeatedly make gratitude lists. I read them daily. During depression, disappointment, or challenge, I read my Gratitude Inventory many times in a day. Gratitude restores my balance and healthy perspective, so I don't get swallowed by negativity. My Gratitude Inventory neutralizes fear and pain.

Don't waste, spill, or squander life's blessings. Capture the good moments on paper. Count them. Remember them. Treasure them. Celebrate the awesome beauty of God's creation. Gratitude is one of your strongest healing powers.

Positive memories bring positive, healing energies into every cell of your body. Positive energies bring their friends. Multiply the positive energy in your life by greedily treasuring every positive moment.

In the following space, write your Gratitude Inventory. Be sure to update it as the weeks go by. Remember, gratitude is a precious ally. There's nothing to do but rejoice and give thanks!

_____

_____

_____

_____

_____

Your Lifetime Treasure Box

Bank your happy memories. Bank them carefully.
You will need to draw upon them in difficult times.
—Judith Larkin Reno, Ph. D.

Count your garden by the flowers,
Never by the leaves that fall.
Count your days by the golden hours,
Don't remember clouds at all.
Count the nights by stars, not shadows.
Count your life by smiles, not tears.
—Unknown

When you are bed-ridden or close to death, your memories gain importance. They are the treasures of your lifetime, belonging only to you. You don't have a future, but you do have a past.

To help during the difficult times, create a Lifetime Treasure Box. Fill it with happy memories from your entire life. Different from your Daily Harvest Necklace or your Gratitude Inventory, your Lifetime Treasure Box spans a lifetime of collected high points and victories. Select your favorite pinnacle memories, such as graduations, weddings, births, or trips.

The memories you retrieve are precious. Treat them with great respect, like valuable jewels. Take them out and polish them. Admire them. Enjoy them often. These are the jewels in your crown.

You may scan your life to harvest memories by regular time periods, for example every five years. Or, you may troll for treasure using developmental periods: infant, toddler, pre-school, grade school, junior high, senior high, young adult, adult, mid-life, senior status.

You may retrieve memories by the houses you lived in; the jobs you had; or the cars you drove. Love relationships may define periods of treasure mining. Some people recall the clothes they wore or popular songs to trigger memories.

You might pull out old photo albums or talk to family members. Ask friends and family what they think your favorite memories are. Their list might delight you!

To find your lifetime treasures, think of your life as a movie with beginning, middle, and end. See the leading actors, villains, and heroes. Who were your mentors and guides in this life? Who did the most to shape you? What were the defining events in your life? Remember happy trips you took, places you visited, historic sites, and locations.

Remember favorite people. Who made you laugh? Whom did you respect? Who loved you the best? Whom did you love the most? Who was a catalyst for growth? Who made you think? List your best friends.

What are the great triumphs and achievements of your life? Note the people and places connected with these times.

Collect your lifetime treasures. Don't waste them. Honor their place in your life. Now is the time to harvest them.

While scouting for treasures, your mind may want to distract you with disappointing memories, resentments, unfulfilled dreams, etc.

These are part of everyone's life experience. Stay focused on happy, victorious memories.

While negative experiences contain wisdom gifts, the focus for your Lifetime Treasure Box is on positive memories. Harvest healing power from your happy memories.

Below, list the great triumphs of your life for your Lifetime Treasure Box:

_____

_____

_____

_____

_____

SWEET TALK

It's a funny thing about life; if you refuse to accept anything but the best, you very often get it.
—Somerset Maugham

Your Word Is Your Power

Your words build the house you live in.
—Hafiz, Thirteenth Century Sufi Poet

Your word is your power to create. It declares the laws of your life. The *Bible* says, "In the beginning was the word." All manifest form emerged out of the word. You create your reality from the power of your word, both spoken and thought.

Be sure your words serve you. Thought is prayer. Whatever you speak repeatedly, you affirm. Remember the Upanishads, "What a man thinks, he becomes."

If you want to be healthy, think of yourself as healthy. Speak of yourself as healthy. Disengage from disease labels. Instead of speaking of your disease, talk about your "condition" or your "diagnosis." Avoid saying, "My disease." Such declaration of ownership reinforces a disease connection in your subconscious mind.

When doctors talk about "cancer," let the word be like water off a duck's back to you. Don't allow society's panic and fear regarding the c-word to enter your consciousness.

Because of society's misplaced emotionalism, avoid using the word, chemo, in talking with friends. Some TV dramas show the way chemo was years ago. They can create deep fear around the treatment. I've heard people say, "I would rather die from cancer than go through chemo." To avoid sensationalism and create dignity instead, refer to chemo as "medicine" or "my treatment."

In my self-talk prior to chemo treatments, I call the chemo "my sweet medicine." I praise and admire its ability to seek and destroy the unwanted cells. I make friends with the treatment. In my thoughts and words, I emphasize chemo's positive qualities.

Once, I overheard patients in the hospital ward discussing their diseases. They were in ferocious competition to see who had the worst disease. It was a classic demonstration of abusing the power of the word. Because of the intense emotion behind their words, they were actually reinforcing their diseases. They were ignorant of the power of their word.

Words are literal. Examine the vibration they set in motion to create your life. Is the energy positive or negative? Finding the correct word demands clarity. Clarity is the first step to manifestation.

When you receive a cancer diagnosis, you may get a "Handicapped" sign to hang in your car for parking spaces close to the door. Be careful not to adopt the handicapped label as part of your identity. Don't begin to fashion your self-concept as disabled. It is a subtle distinction, but one worth noticing. Think of yourself as special and extraordinary, rather than handicapped. Appreciate that God only distributes the most challenging assignments to the strongest Souls.

Constantly be on the alert to translate negative to positive thinking. The word is one of your most powerful healing allies. The wise man once said, "Only talk when it improves the silence."

Sweet Self-Talk

To love oneself is the beginning of a life long romance.
—Oscar Wilde

In the end, all you have is yourself and God. It behooves you to create a great relationship with yourself. Practice talking with yourself sweetly.

Sometimes when you're ill, there's a negative internal script that says, "You did something wrong." When things keep going "wrong," it's easy to become judgmental.

Don't confuse external events with your identity or your value. Monitor your self-talk. Instead of blaming yourself for disease, see that you are a courageous spiritual warrior fighting for Truth through the healing journey. Celebrate yourself as a spiritual hero!

When you give yourself love-lavish, you become your own best friend. You enjoy yourself. You champion and parent yourself. You emphasize the heroic nature of your journey in your self-talk. You self-nurture.

If disappointment comes, name and validate your experience. Let your internal Divine Mother and Father referee and resolve your emotions—the way a healthy parent guides squabbling children to peace. Discuss inner conflicts with your God Self and your Soul.

Hear the unconditionally loving voice of your Soul say, "You did the best you could. There is no blame. You did nothing wrong. You are the perfect child of a loving God. What happened is perfect in its way. It could not have been otherwise. I love and treasure you, just the way you are."

The Soul never berates you, even when suggesting a change in attitude or behavior. Align with your Soul to reframe negative words to positive. When you talk to yourself, be respectful. Use humor to lighten up. Negative self-talk is hurtful.

Peace Pilgrim was an inspiring woman who walked across the country for many years with the single purpose of spreading love. She said, "Good is when you help people. Bad is when you hurt people. Including yourself."

Body-Talk Skills

There are no conditions beyond God's power to heal.
—Judith Larkin Reno, Ph. D.

If part of your body hurts, talk to it. Clearly visualize it and interview it.

Say, Why are you hurting? What do you need from me? How can I help you? Do you need touch? Massage? Water? Exercise? Nutritional supplements? Special food? Heat? Cold? Are you inflamed? Dehydrated? Calcified? Twisted? Queasy? Cramped? What do you need for balance?

Ask the hurting part to light up. What color is it? The color may indicate what your body needs. If it is red, the area may be inflamed and require some cooling blue Light to calm it.

Ask the body-part what color Light it needs to be happy. What color will balance it and erase the pain? Visualize the rainbow. Infuse different rays of color into your body. Which color infusion provides balance? Which color eases the pain? Which color increases your strength?

In your body interview, become microscopic and travel inside the upset area. Notice how the landscape changes as you enter the pain zone. Act like a reporter noticing every detail of the landscape. Describe the "weather." Interview the locals.

Unify with the pain and describe it. What symbol or icon describes the pain? A block of ice? A lightning bolt? A sharp tack? A heavy weight? You can't fix a pain until you can name it.

Dialogue with the pain. Ask what it needs to go away. What has it come to teach you? What must you learn before it will leave? What gift or benefit does it give you?

Body talk involves body listening. After you ask the question, notice what springs to mind. Accept the first thought, image, memory, or feeling as your body's answer. The body often speaks in symbols, like dream symbols. Pay close attention.

The first thought after your question is the body's response. Trust that. You may easily overlook the answer since it often comes in a flash—literally a fraction of a second.

It is your job to decode the answers and learn your body's language. Follow what "feels" right and you will develop a trusting and intimate relationship with your body.

Your body might complain of lack of love, poor circulation, or temperature imbalance. Sometimes the voice will be exhausted and overworked. You must listen closely and remedy whatever you can.

Be proactive in finding remedies. Seek help from experts. Research remedies on the Internet and through reading. Ask friends to help in researching information.

Enlist your body to cooperate with you. Make a deal. For example, say, "I will give you lots of love and Light if you stop cramping on me." Then be sure to feed the body its favorite color of Light and plenty of love throughout the day.

Talk to your body gently like a parent to a beloved child. Tell the body how much you love it. Express how valuable the hurting body part is. Explain that you can't live without it.

Ask your body to normalize. Use the billions of healthy people in the world as a standard to teach your body what "healthy" feels like. Ask your body to copy their model of health and well-being.

Place your hand over the ailing body part. Send healing energy and love through your hand into your body. Sometimes, you can immediately feel it become happy again.

To increase healing, move your hand in a circle over the pain. Use your inhale to drive healing energies deep into the hurt place. Feel God's infinite supply of love and healing pour through your hand into your body. Open yourself to receive God's healing just as a flower opens to the sun. Don't limit the supply of healing you receive.

Inhale God's healing Light deep into the hurt place.

On the exhale, see anything negative, toxic, or unbalanced release from your body. See a dark, soot-like energy lift off your body. Inhale Light. Exhale darkness.

As you advance your daily body talk, commiserate with ailing body parts. Validate the hurt voice, just as a wise parent names and validates the child's journey. Use sweet talk with your body.

For example, say to your kidney, "I notice you are irritable. I don't blame you. You have been overworked lately. Anyone in your position would be angry. Your anger is drawing the line. It's saying, 'No. I won't work any harder.' I appreciate your pain and hard work, dear kidney. However, I need you to be strong and happy for this next treatment. How can we work together so you feel better? What can I do to help you? I'll search the Internet for supplements. I'll call friends and ask for recommendations. I'll change my diet to foods less irritating. I love and cherish you, dear kidney. I will champion your good health and happiness."

Falling asleep at night is an especially fertile zone for healing. As you relax, opening to sleep, your brain is easily hypnotized. Use this time to praise, coach, and cheerlead body parts. Program your body for healing. Visualize and feel your body healed.

For example, tell your bones what a great job they did today. Say, "I see your bone mass increasing every day. Good job! Stay in strong form. I need you. I love you." Visualize them healed—in perfect condition. Send electric white Light to every bone in your body to increase its strength. Feel the Light vibrate in your bones. Get a chart of your bones, so you can visualize them more clearly.

Preparing for radiation or chemo treatments, talk to your body. Explain that a wonderful new medicine is coming to heal you and give you a better life. Ask your body to welcome the medicine as a savior and ally. Invite your body to treat the medicine as an honored guest in your home.

Avoid polarizing in resistance against your medicine. Instead, unify with the treatment through praise and appreciation.

Before stem cell or bone marrow transplant, talk to your bone marrow. Explain that it is about to graduate. It is being replaced, but not because it did anything wrong. On the contrary, because it succeeded in helping you to heal, you now qualify for a transplant. This is a great victory.

Praise your marrow for its strength and perseverance. Explain that help is on the way. New marrow is coming to carry the load. The old marrow is free to graduate, retire, and enjoy a well-deserved rest. Congratulations!

Use body talk to let your catheter know how much you appreciate it. Tell it how grateful you are that it saves you from the pain of needles. Say, "You are a true best friend. I love and honor you for all the help you give me." See your catheter light up as it receives your praise.

As with all of us, the body loves praise. Praise your organs, glands, blood, bones, muscles, nerves, and lymph. Praise every part of your body daily. Praise and body talk are profoundly healing.

CANCER

God alone suffices.
—St. Theresa of Avila

The elephant that is going unnoticed in our societal tent is the national cancer epidemic. Estimates predict 40% of Americans will be diagnosed with cancer. Cancer is the biggest killer of Americans under 75 years old. One of every two men will get cancer in his lifetime. One of every three women will get cancer.

Imagine three jumbo jets full of people crashing every day. That is the number of people who die with cancer, daily. Now, imagine one of the World Trade Twin Towers collapsing every day—that's cancer. Fifteen hundred people die of cancer, daily.

Between the ages of 45 to 64, cancer kills more people than the next three causes of death combined. Clearly, it's time to declare national war on cancer.

In the 1970's President Nixon declared war on cancer. Since then, cancer has increased. The nation has been lulled and distracted. Now is the time to face this national epidemic.

Baby boomers are the largest generation in the history of the US. With their aging, our nation's senior population is burgeoning. By 2025, estimates predict 25% of the population will be seniors. Seniors are prime targets for cancer.

Why is the nation asleep to the cancer epidemic in our midst? We need to declare a serious national war on cancer. We don't need any more elephants in our tents!

Practical Tips While in the Hospital

Pray and tie your camel.
—Arabic Saying

Managing disease requires great personal skill. At a practical level, I learned some useful tricks dealing with the medical world and hospitals. I experienced seven hospitalizations in fifteen months, including eight aggressive chemotherapies, two stem-cell transplants, and twelve surgical procedures. I learned to set my hospital visits up for success.

To facilitate fast healing, I brought many support items. They helped me to normalize and mood-alter when times got tough.

I brought the following items: a brightly colored comforter for my bed; a bulletin board for the wall opposite my bed, where I could display greeting cards and inspirational slogans; my boom box with lots of audio tapes and CD's, including talking tapes, both humorous and inspirational; my VCR/DVD player with videos, including comedies. Since hospital furniture is sparse, I brought a wicker basket to hold my support items and to reduce clutter in the room.

To stay in God alignment, I brought objects to empower my spirit: pictures of saints, Guruji, my Soul Council, family, and friends; my Prayer Team Album; my Prayer Team Phone List; small, four-by-six-inch, picture albums of my daughters' weddings, my grandson's birth, and favorite times with my husband—central motivators in my fight to live.

The small albums are easy to lift. Some days, I experienced profound fatigue. An empty dinner plate was too heavy to lift. I broke numbers of them at home. I wanted photo albums that could serve me on my weak days.

In addition, I brought books; writing materials; my journal; and a calendar, so I could mark time, display victories, and feel progress as I crossed off each day. I brought games to pass the time playing cards, Scrabble, backgammon, etc. Some people bring their laptop computers. However, security can be an issue.

Rather than wear hospital gowns, I dressed in bright, colorful clothes from home. I brought my best shirts to cheer me up, even though I knew they might be damaged by iodine spills and dressing changes from my catheter. The risk was worth the emotional boost to my self-esteem. I brought lots of clothes, since a clean outfit was needed each day for hospital hygiene.

My case was unusual, due to the complications of cryoglobulinemia added to bone cancer combined with a broken back. I had to educate each doctor and nurse who helped me.

The cryoglobulinemia meant if I got the slightest bit cold, my blood could clot and I could experience a life-threatening hemorrhage. I was extremely sensitive to cold and had to keep warm all the time. In addition, the cryo added to my extreme sensitivity to pain—far beyond what a normal person experiences. Since cryo is rare, doctors and nurses needed to have it explained.

At first, I had assumed that doctors and nurses would be prepped regarding my case. After all, they were the experts. They were supposed to take care of me. Right? *Wrong!*

I soon discovered I was in charge of my healing program. If I wanted success, I had to be proactive. I learned to train my team of healers. The exotic nature of my complex diagnosis was so rare, they didn't understand my needs. I had to teach them how to care for me.

Each doctor was a specialist, isolated in his field of specialization. Since they were oncologists, not orthopedic specialists, the doctors easily forgot my broken and dislocated bones. None of them understood my extreme pain and cold sensitivity from the cryo. I constantly had to remind my medical team, both doctors and nurses, of my situation.

Teaching the hospital staff was no easy rigor, since I had seven different doctors and innumerable nurses. In addition, I was often semicomatose due to pain and medications.

To get my needs met in the hospital, I learned to communicate in vivid word-pictures, using concrete images. For example, due to over a year of caustic, aggressive, chemo treatments, I had phlebitis—inflamed veins. In a normal case, blood pressure readings cause little or no pain. In my case, the pressure cuff was excruciatingly painful. To convey the degree of pain I experienced, I asked the nurse to imagine an open, raw flesh wound with a wet rope rubbing across it.

The vivid word-picture not only informed the nurse of my unusual pain condition, but also automatically enlisted her to find a solution. My arms were extremely sore from months of blood pressure readings. Black-and-blue marks and varicose veins delineated the cuff placement. Shifting from an arm to a calf cuff provided some relief.

In addition to using vivid word-pictures to communicate, I created innovative solutions to my many problems. I invented new protocols, designing applications to fit my situation. Then, I trained the doctors and nurses to use them.

None of this was easy. Doctors are not easily led. Medical staff wear mental blinders, thinking there is only one way for treatment. Nurses worried about reprimands if they changed the protocol to help me. With my rare diagnosis, I didn't fit their models.

I learned not to accept their assumptions, to honor my needs, to speak up, to offer suggestions, and to go to the supervisor if necessary. I also learned to be persistent. Problem solving, communication, and enlistment skills were essential to my success.

As a people helper by profession, I was accustomed to giving help. The skills of asking for help were difficult to learn. At first, I was so codependent I didn't want to press my Nurse Call button for fear of disturbing or inconveniencing someone!

Slowly, I learned my entitlement. After all, the staff worked for me. I paid for their services. The staff trained to help me. They wouldn't be there unless they wanted to help me. They were designed to serve me. As with the angels, I disappointed them if I didn't call on their services.

I learned to ask for help in a clear, non-adversarial way. I had to overcome fears of sounding demanding, angry, bitchy, or whiny. Asking for help triggered my victim issues.

Not speaking hospitalese, I wasn't sure of the right "hospital" language. To retain a modicum of dignity and not regress to potty-training days, I quizzed nurses for the best words to use.

During chemo, the digestive tract is the star of the show. Nurses record and measure all the patient's urine and bowel movements. I asked the nurse what language to use when I needed her to take a measurement. She coached me to say, "I need help in the bathroom." Or, "I have a collection." She said the measurement cups are called hats. So, I could also say, "I have a hat to be measured."

Proper language was empowering and liberating. With the right words, I felt comfortable again. The Nurse Call transaction no longer involved personal power or control. I was just part of a team getting a job done. I reframed myself from a victim to an empowered team member.

When mistakes happened—as they will—I didn't take them personally. Instead, my perspective was God-centered. I understood all events as a part of God's perfect plan for me—regardless of negative appearances.

Nurses and nurse's assistants change shifts every eight to twelve hours, not necessarily at the same time. You may have different nurses and assistants every day of your hospital stay, never seeing the same face twice. As a patient, I found the turnover exhausting, especially due to the unusual nature of my case where I had to educate everyone who worked on me.

Even though I was semicomatose and pain-ridden, I made an extra effort to memorize the names of my nurses. I asked each nurse to write her name on my bulletin board. This small handle kept me from falling into depersonalized anonymity and alienation. In addition, I think you get better service if you have a personal connection with each nurse.

Studies show that happy people feel in control of their lives. Hospitalization can make you feel a radical loss of control. Being bed-bound, hooked to an IV, and having to ask for everything do not contribute to your feeling empowered.

While in the hospital, do everything you can to empower yourself. Make everything pleasant for yourself, to the extent possible.

Hospital studies indicate that the smallest act of personal empowerment improves psychological well-being. Even making menu choices is empowering! Choosing and wearing my own clothes added to my healthy sense of control.

I planned a daily personal agenda to empower myself. Each evening, I asked the nurses about my schedule for the next day. In free time, I scheduled audio tapes, videos, reading, cards, games, and phone calls. These personal "rewards" balanced my pleasure/pain seesaw and gave me a healthy sense of control. Each day, I looked forward to my treats, despite the medical rigors.

Numbers of interruptions in a hospital day can undermine your healthy sense of control. I remember trying to watch a video movie and counting fifteen interruptions by hospital staff in a ninety-minute period. I had to learn a completely new skill of living without privacy or continuity.

Whenever I started a personal project, I did some self-talk preparing myself for interruptions. I realized all these people worked for me. Each one was there to help me. Each one was fighting to save my life. The interruptions were not personal or impolite. It was my job to welcome each interruption with love and gratitude—knowing it was bringing me closer to my goal of healing.

Prior to my illness, I associated hospitals with fear, having heard endless horror stories in the media of sponges sewed inside people and healthy organs mistakenly removed. After spending time in hospitals as a patient, I have the reverse view. Each time I was hospitalized, the staff literally saved my life. I see doctors and nurses as heroic, compassionate, and highly skilled. Modern medicine offers miracles, especially in acute care situations.

There are more angels in hospitals than anywhere I've ever been. To be in a hospital is a mystical field day. The angels congregate in response to the need for healing. God goes where God is needed. Angelic presence is almost everywhere you look. Opportunities abound for making new angel friends.

Many of the angels are of the blue ray. Love and healing pours out of their eyes. They stand in a horseshoe around the patient's head and shoulders. If you are in a hospital, as either a patient or a visitor, don't miss the opportunity to mingle with these divine beings!

Sun Lover

Before sunlight can shine through a window, the blinds must be raised.
—American Proverb

The sky is daily bread for the eyes.
—Ralph Waldo Emerson

I don't usually sit in the sun long—just enough to balance my pituitary, the master gland that aligns the body with healing. While I receive its grace, I talk to the sun, praising and honoring its powers. The sun is the life-giver. Without the sun, life on earth would extinguish.

I consciously absorb the sun's vital force into every atom of my body. As I feel the sun deliciously warming my skin, I luxuriate in the intimacies of the wind running his fingers through my hair.

What an act of cosmic love it is when Sun and I meet unobstructed. He is an ardent lover who travels 93 million miles for our meeting!

The sun actually breathes. Every six minutes it expands, inhaling. Six minutes later, it exhales—actually contracting. To me, the sun is a living friend.

Trapped inside the hospital, I felt deprived of my great joy of sun-sitting. I learned to ask nurses if I could sit in the sun for a few minutes each day. Some hospitals help you find a way.

Otherwise, you might want to enjoy a sunbath ritual sitting in your window. Or, give yourself a revitalizing sun-treatment in your meditation.

When you're sick, you may become touch-deprived. In my case, I was in too much pain to enjoy human touch. My Sun Lover really helped!

Dolphins Who Heal

Because all is one, I know that I am part of all that is. As I travel up my God Ladder, I reach my Higher Self. From my divine side, I have access to infinite supply, intelligence, resource, and healing. They are my birthright.
—Judith Larkin Reno, Ph. D.

I was in my second stem-cell transplant. After receiving caustic chemo-treatments for fifteen months, my veins and mucosa were highly inflamed.

The chemo attacks fast-growing cancer cells. However, it can't distinguish between a cancer cell and other fast-growing cells, such as hair, the mucosal lining of the mouth, or the digestive tract.

Therefore, during and for weeks after the high-dose chemo of stem-cell replacement, as the medicine does its job, hair falls out and the mucosa disintegrates.

The lining of the mouth develops lesions and burns that feel like razor blades every time you breathe, swallow, or eat. Eating with razor blades in your mouth is no fun. It could take me hours to get through a meal with all the pain-pauses.

During a meditation on how to deal with the pain, a dolphin appeared and offered to help. I remembered that dolphins regenerate their skin and mucosa instantaneously when they are scratched. No one has figured out how they do it. It is quite amazing to watch.

Grateful for help, I invoked the dolphins and their instant ability to regenerate mucosa. I visualized healthy, smiling dolphins, swimming in pods inside my mouth, rectum, colon, and anywhere I had a scratch.

In my condition, the tiniest scratch was not only disproportionately painful, but also life-threatening. Without stem cells to make disease-fighting white cells, my immune system was down to zero.

Everywhere the dolphins swam, they aligned with the cells of my body, teaching them the secret healing, regeneration technique. The dolphin's alignment felt like rhythm entrainment.

For example, if you put five grandfather clocks in a room with pendulums swinging at varying rates, by morning they all realign and beat at the highest vibration. The dolphins provided a similar rhythm entrainment. They taught my cells to vibrate at cell-regeneration rate.

My cells imitated the dolphins' modeling. With the dolphins' assistance, I felt some immediate relief. I healed rapidly.

When the pain attacks were at their worst, I called upon the sweet, smiling dolphins as my allies. They were joyful to be called to help.

Baldness Brings Good Luck!

I learn, whatever state I may be in, therein to be content.
—Helen Keller

When a flat, yellow-gold dandelion goes to seed, its shaggy mane transforms. Not only the dandelion's color changes, but also its shape.

Magically, golden dandelion locks achieve senior status, transforming into downy, gray, silk hair. With more magic, the new coif morphs its silky spines into a hair-spiked ball, the size of a marshmallow. The dandelion is a master of shape-shifting—from its youthful goldilocks to its ancient hoary Afro.

If you blow on this ancient dandelion head, a diaspora of soft spider hairs flies off in every direction. Nothing remains but a succulent stem—sporting a round, white knob of spittle daub on top.

If you blow hard enough, you can blow all the hairs off in one try. It is said that this balding ritual brings good luck.

People are always trying to rub my "chemo-cut" baldhead for good luck. They say there is a custom in the East to rub the Buddha's baldhead for luck.

Could it be that shape-shifting into baldness brings good luck? Now, there's a reframe!

Cancer Offers Closure

Think nothing else but that God ordains all, and
where there is no love, put love, and you will draw out love.
—St. John of the Cross

Everyone gets to die. Not everyone gets to say good-bye. The good news about a cancer diagnosis is you often have enough time for the comfort of closure.

My friend Kent died of prostate cancer. In his last year, he wrote his autobiographical summary for his memorial service. He had a chance to sum up his life and to reflect.

He assessed his victories and challenges. Then, he told what he would have changed. Kent was a well-known chemist, so he had many career victories. His challenges were those of juggling career, marriage, family, and friends—without stress and with enough time for each. He would have changed his relationship with family and friends, spending more time with them and less on his career.

Kent wrote letters to each of his daughters and his wife of thirty-four years. In the letters, he stated what he admired about each loved one. He talked about what each one taught him. Then, he said what he wished he had done better. For example, he told his wife Lana that he wished he had changed more diapers as a young father.

These letters helped diffuse the anger that is a natural part of the grief process. They helped each member of Kent's family say good-bye.

In my case, when I was so close to death some of the ministers I had trained held a prayer service for me in a nearby park where I had enjoyed hiking. They taped their testimonials for me to hear.

It was shocking and glorious to hear their love for me. I knew how deeply I loved them, but I never realized the degree of love they had for me. Nor, had I realized the impact I had on their lives. Listening to the tape was like being at my own funeral, with all the benefits of still being alive! After the "funeral," I felt the privilege of my ongoing life as if it were a second life.

In the time between diagnosis and death, cancer can offer a rare opportunity to review your life. You can make peace with friends, family, and memories. You can prepare for death, legally, financially, and emotionally.

Whether you live or die, this time is an opportunity to wrap up the loose ends and put a bow on your life.

PAIN MANAGEMENT

In your hour of adversity, be not without hope,
For crystal rain falls from black clouds.
—Persian Poem

When you're on the bottom looking up, you have the best
perspective.
—Sharon Stone, Actress

When I feel the heat, I see the Light.
—Senator Everett Dirksen

The Observer Mouse Gets Distance from the Pain

You can observe a lot by watching.
—Yogi Berra, Baseball Player

The pain is so great it becomes a ferocious tiger. The tiger has my head in his mouth. We struggle but there is no way out for me. It is hopeless. So, I totally surrender.

At the moment of my surrender, earthly reality becomes the thinnest of veils. It is the same fabric as dreams—filmy and ethereal like cheese-cloth.

A little mouse appears by my side. He chews a hole through the cheese-cloth fabric of life. Together, we jump through the hole into another reality, free from pain. Suddenly, I realize we have penetrated the veil of earthly life and left the human condition.

Outside earthly consciousness, the mouse and I find ourselves on a stage. We are standing beside a giant movie screen. My Guides say, "This is the Screen of Consciousness on which the events of your life appear."

The tiny mouse and I take a front row seat. He curls his tail like a parasol over his head as he enjoys his luxurious, velvet cushion. Together, we watch the movie of my life. We see Judith wrestling with her pain, struggling with the tiger.

We are not involved with them. Instead, we observe characters in a movie while we munch our popcorn. As a spectator, I am free from their drama.

Eventually, I get bored watching them. I float far away into the peaceful void of the cosmos. I become the space between the stars.

Released from the pleasure/pain trance of earthly existence, I no longer confuse my identity with my life. I am not my pain. The pain is far away.

However, before I float into the embrace of my cosmic family, I give my sweet Observer Mouse a hefty piece of cheese.

Bi-Level Viewing

*The question is not how to escape the pain, but what to do
while it's hurting.*
—Judith Larkin Reno, Ph. D.

I am happiest when I don't take my life too seriously. My point of power is when I participate in and observe my life, at the same time. If I put some distance between "me" and my life, I have breathing space. When I'm both the movie and the audience of my life, I am free.

Divine-witnessing my life, I'm not trapped by events. This double view creates detachment from pain. If I maintain the equanimity of standing outside my life observing it, while simultaneously passionately living it, I receive the most joy. I don't confuse the events of my life with my identity.

As my dear friend Russ Phelps says, "Practice high involvement and low attachment." Bi-level viewing ensures that I'm unattached to earthly ups and downs. I stop obsessing on my life. My identity expands to include God.

Through my divine witness, I see my life in the context of eternity and infinity—my refuge. I am no longer a victim. My God-link returns.

My personal life, like movies, is destined to dissolve. By contrast, the impersonal Screen of Consciousness behind transitory events endures. It is permanent and universal, beyond the earthly light show.

The Screen is untouched by the images played on it. Movies of fire, flood, earthquake, or tornado leave the Screen undamaged. It is unmoved and undiminished by pain or violence.

Bi-level viewing of my life empowers me with the larger perspective—beyond pain. My divine witness opens me to a detached, objective view beyond my personal experience. My view expands to include God.

Divine Witnessing

Pain contracts your attention. Spiritual witnessing expands it.
—Judith Larkin Reno, Ph. D.

Suffering has no divine witness.
—Judith Larkin Reno, Ph. D.

Christian mysticism says, "Enlightenment is being in the world, but not of it." With divine witnessing, you see your body, emotions, and mind as separate from you, although you fully experience each of them. They are yours to manage. However, they are not your identity. You are in the world, but you are also simultaneously beyond it.

Your primary identification is with your divine side. Your God Self sees today's challenge in the context of eons and vast universes. By contrast, personal problems are tiny and temporary.

When you see through God Glasses and Soul Vision, the struggle drops away. Everything is OK, just as it is. Soon the earthly movie will change to the next scene. A new plot will emerge. At the end of the movie, you will leave the theater. There is an exit.

The Sacred Now of divine witnessing contains both your personal present and your impersonal eternity. It references both your earthly and divine sides, integrating them.

To spiritually witness requires that you don't judge yourself, others, life, or God. You can discern, name, assess, evaluate, and choose. However, you must not judge. Divine witnessing is impartial and detached from your personal ego, fears, or desires.

Fighting disease, you can lose your divine witness. Your stomach churns with nausea. Your emotions avalanche with fear. Your mind obsesses on the future.

During challenges, practice anchoring in your divine witness. When you feel helpless, ask God to help you. For an instant, shift your view from inside events to seeing through God's eyes. Call upon your Infinite Supply.

You can't move a pain-rock if you are standing on it! Your leverage comes when you jump off the rock. Using your divine witness moves you off the pain-rock. The power and perspective of your divine witness give you leverage to move your pain.

Divine witnessing shifts your attention from fixating on pain. Your divine witness unchains your identity from pain.

Invite your divine witness to co-star in your new buddy movie. I'll even lend you my Observer Mouse to keep you company!

Detachment Skills

Sometimes I hear God shouting at me, "Get out of the way and let me in!"
—Judith Larkin Reno, Ph. D.

In the film *Lawrence of Arabia*, Lawrence holds his hand over a candle flame until the flesh starts burning. His friend asks if his hand hurts. Lawrence answers, "Yes. But the trick is not to mind."

Learn to dissociate in a healthy way. When pain comes, step into your divine Time/Space Machine. Peel off from your body and go to the moon. Divine witness your crisis from 1,000 years in the future or from another planet. Use your God Glasses and Soul Vision.

Buddha taught detachment from earthly events. Buddhist monks chant, *"I am not my body. I am not my emotions. I am not my mind. I am that which is greater."* Memorize this chant. Use it.

The great East Indian saint Sri Nisargadatta says, "Your power is in your detachment." When negative events come, let them roll over you. Put up your firewall. Stay uninvolved. Disengage from earthly levels. Stand outside events. Unhook from intense emotions. Find the untouched place inside.

Ride Kuan Yin's dragons of detachment up your God Ladder to your divine side. Take a vacation from earth's challenges. Use your divine spectator to create distance from events.

To cultivate detachment, once a day wash your face with an ice-cold washcloth. Before the shock of the cold, anchor your identity in your divine witness. Say, "I am not my body. I am God, Goodness, the Infinite Divine."

Inhale and concentrate your will. Master Morya specializes in willpower and focused concentration. Call on him to help you stay focused.

On the exhale, proceed with the cold washcloth while maintaining your detached God-witness. Be unmoved by the cold. Run it down through your body and out into the earth. Maintain your detached viewpoint, witnessing as the cold moves through you.

This exercise strengthens your spiritual muscles for detachment. When I do this exercise, I often think of Kathryn Hepburn. She swam in the cold river every morning during New York winters. When asked why she subjected herself to such discipline, she replied, "It builds character."

Practice seeing pain from a distance. Dump the pain in the Holy Fields of Non-Caring. The Field of Detachment is your salvation. Sometimes, it's healthy not to care. After your coldness exercise, wear your "I don't care" tee shirt.

To detach from the suffering game, use the following wisdom: If it looks as if there isn't enough (life, love, money, health, medicine, time, etc.), then you are trying too hard. Relax. Breathe. Let go. Smile. Stop trying so hard. Embrace the Sacred Now.

Remember the words of the French maxim. "Things are never as good or bad as they seem."

Naming Skills

When you name something, you have power over it.
—Native American and East Indian Traditions

Naming skills are the foundation of bi-level witnessing. When you name, you witness your life. The part of you that names is God. Naming brings you closer to God. It is a form of justice. Naming returns you to the Sacred Now.

In the subject/object distinction of naming, you separate your True Identity from the pain. Returning to your True Self, you create sacred space, detached perspective, and objectivity.

To name, you must be present in both your earthly and divine levels, simultaneously. Bi-level witnessing ensures non-attachment and decreases suffering.

Throughout the day, name your experience as if you are a news commentator, dispassionately observing the events of your life. Naming is not blaming. Rather, naming is clear-seeing and discernment without judgmentalness. Objectively, name both the "good" and "bad" experiences. Say, "This feels good. That hurts."

Until you can describe your pain specifically, you can't diagnose and heal it. You can't enlist others to help. Doctors and nurses can serve you better, if you have naming skills to describe your pain. Family and friends understand your journey better if you accurately name it.

Name your pain. Is it physical, emotional, mental, or spiritual? Characterize your pain in concrete, vivid, physical images and word-pictures. Create a physical icon or symbol for your pain. Objectifying pain gives you power over it.

Through four years of constant acute pain, I got up-close-and-personal with it. Like Eskimos with one hundred names for snow, I catalogued many names for my pain.

For example, one pain felt like rats eating my bones. Another felt like red-hot pokers shooting through my body. The everyday chronic background ache was always there, like the roar of a giant tanker-truck engine. It was difficult to hear anything above the roar.

Some days, when the pain flared out of control, I had a rampaging bull-elephant in my tent. Other days, I lay flat as a pancake under my pain elephant. All my energy deflated in profound fatigue.

Then, there was the emotional pain of chemical cries, sudden sadness, hopelessness, fear, and anger. I saw my false beliefs of lack-and-limit thinking feeding my negative emotions. Did I trust God or disease? Confronting my spiritual trust-issues, there were many chiropractic adjustments for my Soul!

Naming skills differ for each level of your being: physical, emotional, mental, and spiritual.

In physical witnessing, you notice and describe body parts that experience pain. Also, identify how the pain affects your five senses: sight, sound, taste, touch, and smell.

When you witness your emotional body, you may hear, "I feel sad, angry, or frightened." These are the basic, most common shadow emotions. During self-interview, you don't need to take action. Just name and validate your emotions without judgment—like an empathetic Divine Parent. Negative emotions need conscious naming and validation to resolve.

Naming is a form of validation. You care enough about your emotion to discern its name. When you listen to your emotion, it feels valued and respected. Internal tension relaxes. Naming is a healing confessional that downloads stress from your body.

Emotions exist to serve you in some way. Negative emotions carry gifts of learning. When you erase emotions without witnessing them, they can't serve you.

When you witness your mind, notice how pain affects your thoughts. You may notice negative, self-limiting thoughts, such as, "Life is impossible." "I'll never make it." "God betrayed me." You can't change a false belief until you name it. Then, you can transmute negative to positive thinking.

When you witness your spiritual bodies, you transcend the dualized, lower three levels: physical, emotional, and mental. Naming your spiritual experience moves you from limited earthly facts to infinite divine Truth. It opens you to miracles.

When you name your spiritual experience, it is usually positive, even if you are learning difficult earthly lessons. However, disease can activate a crisis of faith. Keep alert to resolve your issues with God. See the chapter "Reinvent Your God." Talk to your priest, minister, rabbi, imam, or cleric when doubts arise.

You need God now more than ever. Naming returns you to objectivity and the Sacred Now. From the Sacred Now, you can access God's infinite healing, refuge, and supply.

Pain Dialogue

Pain is a grief experience. You are dealing with loss and problem solving.
—Judith Larkin Reno, Ph. D.

Ninety million Americans live in chronic physical pain. That's 30% of the nation! Whether your pain is physical, emotional, mental, or spiritual there are styles of engagement that can be productive. Here are some strategies I used to combat pain.

In pain wars, you must assess the enemy. Pain dialogue helps you ascertain pain's patterns, strengths, and weaknesses. Using pain dialogue, you name and describe your pain so you can resolve it.

Pain Dialogue

- **Invite your Soul** to witness your pain dialogue.
- **Unify** with the pain, while simultaneously sustaining your detached Soul-witness.
- **Witness and name** the pain to identify its patterns.
- **Identify** the pain's physical, emotional, mental, and spiritual components. Dialogue with one level at a time.
- **Find an object, image, or icon that symbolizes** the pain, e.g., block of ice; hell-fire; bees stinging. Create a vivid, concrete, physical word-picture describing the pain.
- **Personify** the pain. Imagine the pain as a person. Who would it be? What does it look like? Is it male or female? Old or young?

A witch? A gremlin? A tyrant? A cripple? A martyr? A victim? A pitiful orphan? A critic? A judge? A movie character?

- **Give the pain a nickname**—human, animal, or an object. Alternatively, you may ask the pain-person its name.
- **Dialogue with your pain-person** to gain insight and information.
- **Identify the issues of the conflict** between you and the pain. Explain that you're not comfortable with its affliction. List the ways the pain hurts and hinders you. What does it keep you from doing?
- **Find conflict resolution.** Ask the pain-person what it needs for resolution. What has the pain come to teach you? What must you learn before it will leave? How must you change? What will replace the pain when it has gone?
- **Work at problem solving.** What will resolve this pain? Each pain is different. Open your thinking to new solutions. You may want to expand your healing team. Brainstorm solutions from different perspectives on your God Ladder.
- **Take responsibility** for dealing with your pain.
- **Honor your pain** as your teacher.
- Keep dialoguing until you **find the gift of wisdom** in the pain.

Invite your Soul to witness your pain dialogue. Your Soul is your Divine Mother. She protects you, ensuring balance in your pain dialogue. She is unconditionally loving, wise, and comforting. While your Soul may encourage you to change, she never judges you.

Ask her to name and validate your pain. Your Soul might say, "I understand your pain. Of course you feel outraged. Anyone would feel angry given your circumstance." A simple Soul-witness can restore sanity and objective perspective.

Use your Soul-witness throughout your pain dialogue. She creates distance from the pain so it doesn't swallow you. Soul Vision provides an expanded, objective, divine view.

Unify with the pain, while simultaneously sustaining your Soul-witness. By going into the pain instead of away from it, the pain often dissipates. Become one with your pain. Experience it totally. Momentary indulgence allows you to assess the pain.

Witness and name the pain. Like a skilled investigative reporter, notice all its qualities and characteristics. Become "Detective Dog" as you describe the pain in detail. Is it acute? Chronic? Sharp? Is it background pain? Is it all-devouring, consuming all your attention? Write your list of describers so they won't slip from memory.

Use all five senses to name the pain. If the pain were a color, what color would it be? If it were a sound, what voice would it have? What smell, taste, and touch describe the pain?

What patterns does the pain have? What triggers the pain? What time of day, temperature, people, events, foods, or activities trigger the pain? How does the pain affect your daily living?

In witnessing your pain, identify what organ, gland, or nerve center the pain most affects. Which chakra does the pain invade, over-stimulate, or drain?

Identify the physical, emotional, mental, and spiritual components of the pain. You may need to interview them separately.

- See "Body-Talk Skills" to focus on your physical pain.
- Does the physical pain bring emotional friends, such as fear, anger, or sadness? To reframe negative emotions, reference "Gifts of Negative Emotions" and "Reframe Pain to Power."
- Are there any false beliefs that increase your pain? The chapter on "False Beliefs" helps you to identify your cognitive distortions.
- To heal spiritual pain, review "Krishna's Pearls of Wisdom," "Your God Glasses," "Your Truth Compass," and "Who is Your God?"

Create a vivid, concrete, physical image that symbolizes your pain. What material icon or object represents your pain? A block of cement? A Mack truck? Quicksand? Find a visual image of the pain.

Personify your pain in a clear, dramatic human image. See your pain as a person. Anthropomorphizing the pain further separates you from it. Personifying also deepens your interview.

If your pain were a person, who would it be? What would it look like? How would you costume your pain? What colors does it wear? Would it be male or female? Young or old? Quiet or noisy? How does it walk? Notice its voice. How do you feel when you look into its eyes? What person from your childhood does the figure suggest?

To create your pain character, you may draw from film, literature, TV, history, and people you have known. Exaggerate your pain-person's costume as if s/he were in a cartoon or horror movie.

Create a nickname for your pain. Ask the pain-person its name. What does it want you to call it? If the pain were your child, what would you name it? The nickname may be an object, animal, or a human name. When the pain reoccurs, mentally note, "That's Ole Harry." Or, "Here comes the Mack truck." Objectivizing pain creates distance from it.

Dialogue with the pain-person as if it were a separate individual. After your question, notice the first thought, symbol, image, memory, or feeling that goes through your mind. That is the pain's answer. It's your job to decode its meaning.

Pain dialogue is similar to your skill of physical body-talk. Both have the goal of healing. Pain dialogue goes deeper than body talk. You can use pain dialogue to interview your physical, emotional, mental, and spiritual bodies.

To focus and intensify your dialogue, put your hand over the affected area of your body. Rub in a circle over the painful part to increase rapport and draw out conversation.

Review the section on "Shadow Interview" to deepen your self-dialogue.

Identify the issues of your conflict with pain. Tell the pain how uncomfortable it makes you feel. Explain how pain interferes with your life.

Direct your pain dialogue to resolution. Ask the pain for solutions. Ask, "How must I change for you to feel your job is done?" Is the solution physical, emotional, mental, or spiritual?

Gain insight into what the pain has come to teach you. Ask, "What do you want from me?" "What must I learn before you will leave?" "Who will replace you?" Often pain won't leave until you learn what it has come to teach you.

Work at problem solving. What will resolve this pain? The process of problem solving unfolds with each new day. You may need physical therapy, better diet, more exercise, more sleep, better sanitation, different medication, a new doctor, a second medical opinion, a pain specialist, alternative or complementary medicine, a naturopath, an acupuncturist, a masseuse, energy medicine, Reiki healing, colonics, a chiropractor, a psychologist, a minister, a support group, or a prayer partner.

Oncologists are specialists. Outside their limited field, they may not know how to solve your pain problem. Open your thinking to new solutions. You may want to expand your healing team. Remember, you are in charge of your healing.

Take responsibility for dealing with your pain. In your Soul Contract, you chose pain to learn something. By acknowledging responsibility, you retrieve your personal power. You are no longer a victim.

Honor your pain. Never judge it wrong. It is here to serve you. Listen to it speak as an honored guest in your home. Invite the pain to tea where you can entertain and interview it. Out of these alliances, you gain knowledge about how the pain works, what it values, and what it wants from you. Let the pain teach you.

Honoring pain as your teacher helps you to respect and reframe it. You no longer see pain as the enemy. Rather, the pain is an ally serving your awakening.

Find the gift of wisdom in the pain. Once you discover what the pain has come to teach you, you usually are home free. The wisdom gift transmutes pain to power.

These pain dialogue skills shine the Light of consciousness on your pain. You can't manage pain effectively until you have taken its measure.

Strategies for Unruly Pain

The good thing about pain is that we forget it.
Otherwise, there would be no siblings!
—Joseph Simpson, Mountain Climber, *Touching the Void*

Some pain is unrelenting, ravenous, and devouring. Unruly pain is beyond teamwork and dialogue. You need additional strategies to keep the pain from running your life.

Strategies for Unruly Pain

- **Use pain medication immediately** when the pain begins, especially with long-term, acute situations. Don't let the pain gain standing and momentum.
- **Detach** from the pain.
- **Distract** yourself from pain with other activities.
- **Banish** the pain.
- **Create a peaceful co-existence** agreement with the pain, like a business **merger**. Accept the pain as part of your life. Stop resisting it.

Pain creates neural pathways in the brain. Like a trail in the forest, the more you walk on a pain-path, the wider and more defined it becomes. With increased use, the pain capacity of neural pathways increases.

However, if you don't use the pain-path, shortly it disappears. To decrease neural pathways carrying pain, **it is important to stop pain early**.

Pain is like a locomotive. If you let it gather steam, it gains speed and power. Its momentum can be difficult to stop. Deal with pain immediately. Don't let it roll over you.

Thankfully, today's medical schools teach palliative care—especially for end-of-life and acute-pain situations. If you choose pharmaceutical support, medicate early—especially in the case of serious illness.

There is no moral judgment in medicating your pain. This is not a time for stoic asceticism or false spiritualizing. God works through the medication as well as the meditation. Both extremes—addiction to drugs or stiff-willed avoidance of medicine—can be inappropriate and unbalanced.

Normalizing yourself through legitimate pain relief does not mean you will become a drug addict. The medication returns you to baseline ordinary consciousness. It doesn't get you high.

Studies done on patients using morphine to relieve extreme pain show a different biochemistry from addicts looking for a high. While there is a titration period in detoxing from any drug, patients with legitimate, acute pain generally don't become addicted to palliative care.

Follow your doctor's advice. In serious, life-threatening illness, you may be surprised by the freedom you have in choosing pain medication.

Depression and anxiety are normal accompaniments to serious illness. Effective medications are available today that were not on the market just a few years ago. Antidepressants may take two to six weeks before they take effect. Search to find the right medication or combination of medications for your situation. When you stop these meds, they often need titration under your doctor's supervision. Therefore, unlike many medicines, there is a time factor involved.

In addition to pharmaceutical support, you can retrain neural pathways in your brain by using mind control. When pain appears, go somewhere else. Use detachment and distraction to outwit the pain.

This is different from repression. In repression, you never identify the pain. You pretend it doesn't exist. You live in a false reality. With detachment and distraction skills, you acknowledge the pain, but choose to direct your thoughts elsewhere.

To strengthen detachment, use your Time/Space Machine. Go up your God Ladder for refuge. See the chapters on "Divine Witnessing," "Detachment Skills," and "Dances with Elephants" for further help with detachment.

Distract your mind from pain. Since the mind can only concentrate on one thing at a time, the pain can't reach you if you think about something else. Develop a lightning-fast response at the first hint of pain. Immediately replace the pain with a positive affirmation, e.g., "Healing is coming now."

Create a team of replacements to distract your mind. For example, think about your breathing. Call upon your Soul Council. See their faces. Repeat their names. Feel each one's presence. Develop refuge with particular saints and heroes. Visit them in your mind. Review "Your Gratitude Inventory," "Your Daily Harvest Necklace," and "Your Lifetime Treasure Box." These are powerful allies.

See "The Boston Elephant Ballet" for more help using distraction to dance with your pain elephant. Have a handy battalion of distractions so when pain appears you have an instant, rehearsed response to combat it.

Sometimes, you must **banish** pain from your Kingdom. Banishment works best with painful emotions or false beliefs, but it also has an effect on physical pain. Banishment requires the utmost willpower, concentration, and follow-through discipline.

To prepare for banishment, use the "Manifestation Technique" in the next section.

When you are ready to banish a particular pain from your Kingdom, be sure to have a bouncer standing beside you. Archangel Michael loves this job. He is a powerful, mighty warrior—known for his strength in battle. A spiritual commando, he loves a good fight. He eats nails for breakfast! Call him. Ask him to "bounce" the pain for you.

Call the pain by name. For example, say, "In God's name, I banish Sorrow from my Kingdom from this day forward!" Imagine a humanized form of sorrow approaching you. Maybe she's dressed in black, shedding ashes as she walks in a stoop-shouldered, slow pace. Exaggerate and dramatize the anthropomorphized behavior and form of the pain.

See battalions of Protector Angels surrounding you in every dimension—walking before you, behind you, to your left and right, above and below you. These are fighter, protector, and defender angels. Feel their mighty protective power. They are champion fighters—the special ops of the God Force. They will keep you safe.

Shout to Sorrow, "Be gone! Never return here! I command Archangel Michael to banish you now!" Watch Archangel Michael escort Sorrow outside the walls of your Kingdom. See the two of them disappear into the horizon.

See the gates of your Kingdom slam shut. Feel the mighty walls of your Inner Kingdom shielding and defending you. You are now impervious to sorrow.

Use your breath to expel physical, emotional, and mental pain. With a firm exhale, shout, "You can't stay here. Be gone!" Focused, intentional breath helps dissolve the pain into nothingness. Push, push, and push the pain out of your body.

You must be vigilant after you banish the pain. Typically, it will try to re-enter. When training a puppy to stay off the sofa, you have to repeat your training until the puppy learns. Similarly, persevere in banishing the pain and eventually it will learn it cannot enter your space.

Another strategy, which is the opposite of banishment, can also work to gain dominion over pain. Try merging with the pain. You used unification earlier to interview pain. Merger is slightly different. **Merger involves a peaceful co-existence agreement** with the pain. It is like a business deal.

In merger, you totally accept the pain as part of your Now. Be present with the pain. Stop resisting it. Let the pain in. Inhale. Exhale. Relax. Lovingly observe the pain without judgment. Become one with it. As you unify with it, you may feel it soften and dissolve. You are taking the polarization out of the pain, becoming allies rather than enemies.

Figure out a way the two of you can live in the same body, like roommates sharing the same home. Ask the pain for ways you can live together in peaceful co-existence.

Mix and match strategies to relieve pain. Over time, you will create a truce or resolution to your pain battle. Learning how to live with pain elephants in your tent is not easy!

Manifestation Technique

Argue for your limitations and sure enough, they're yours.
—Richard Bach

This powerful manifestation technique can be applied to heal every area of your life.

Manifestation Technique

- **Deservability.** Reach clear, unshakable conviction that you deserve freedom from the particular pain. Ask yourself honestly, "Do I deserve freedom from this pain?" Remember, you are a perfect child of a loving God. Claim your deservability.

- **Unify with Infinite Supply.** Claim the Truth of your infinite healing, intelligence, and supply in God Source. Say, "I am one with God's infinite power, now."
- **Visualization.** Clearly see every detail of your new life without pain. Use multisensory awareness. See, feel, hear, taste, and know yourself pain-free. Unify totally with your desired state. Love what you are seeking. See and experience it done!
- **Claim.** Despite appearances, affirm and command yourself free from pain. Say, "I am now pain-free! Thank you God. And so it is." Know the power of your word to create.
- **Surrender.** Release your claim into God's infinite healing power, love, and wisdom.
- **Gratitude.** Feel supreme joy and gratitude for the healing gifts God is bringing to you. Experience your healing as already accomplished.

DANCES WITH ELEPHANTS

Our truest life is when we are in our dreams awake.
—Thoreau

Dance the dream awake.
—Native American Indian

Like the movie *Dances with Wolves,* dancing with pain elephants can be dangerous. Pain can rob your will to live, your sanity, and your Soul. Use the following elephant dance-steps to tame the wild beast.

During pain assaults, you need immediate support. You may not have much energy to read. When pain increases, your window of concentration decreases. These healing lists provide quick, easy access to help.

These **Elephant Dances** are your **mightiest healing lists**, designed for heavy lifting on dark days. Vivid word-pictures and focused slogans cut through brain-fog. High intensity, quick-relief remedies help you dance with your pain elephant.

Use the healing lists like an oracular deck of cards. Close your eyes and run your finger down the list. Notice where your finger stops. That entry is your guide to dancing with your pain elephant. Take its wisdom.

Throw all your concentration into the healing recommendation. Break the pain trance. Praise yourself for every pain-break you create.

In addition to emergency pain management, use the healing lists as food for thought and meditation. They strengthen your spirit to fight pain and disease. Memorize favorite phrases.

Readers describe bringing *Elephants in Your Tent* to chemo and medical procedures. The Elephant Dances help you manage pain, fear, and resistance.

Read the healing lists in bits and snippets throughout the day to keep your love-tank full. They'll also get you through the night, when there is no other support team available.

These power-packed Elephant Dances are constant companions. Read and re-read them to keep pace with your pain elephant. You might even take the lead in a great new dance!

- **The Brazilian Elephant Samba**—A passionate engagement, done belly-to-belly, to *Face Your Fear and Pain,* especially when dealing with needles and medical procedures.
- **The Boston Elephant Ballet**—Elegant choreography to *Distract Your Mind from Pain* and trip the light fantastic.
- **The Texas Elephant Line-Dance**—A country-style promenade to *Work with Pain* and keep your pain in line.
- **The Argentine Elephant Tango**—A fast-moving chase to *Outsmart the Pain* and use your partner's power to your advantage.

Let the humor of dancing with your pulchritudinous pachyderm lighten your load. May terpsichorean delights unfold. May you dance free!

The Brazilian Elephant Samba—Face Your Fear and Pain

I'm so paranoid, I think the people driving ahead of me are
following me the long way around.
—Richard Allen

Just because I'm not paranoid doesn't mean they're not
following me.
—Bumper Sticker

He who has been bitten by a snake is suspicious of a rope.
—Hebrew Expression

FEAR stands for false energy appearing as real.
—Tony Robbins

Fear expense: Fear is not worth my energy expenditure.
—Judith Larkin Reno, Ph. D.

Fear is when you're not looking at your God connection.
—Judith Larkin Reno, Ph. D.

There is appropriate, healthy fear. And, there is disproportional, unhealthy fear. Healthy fear signals a need for caution or more information. Unhealthy fear signals run-away, out-of-control, self-defeating, toxic emotions.

It is normal to get nervous around needles, especially after you've experienced several medical procedures. However, fear can increase and devour your life, unless you stay alert. The instant you notice disproportionate fear, take action to resolve it. Use the Elephant Samba to fortify yourself for needles and medical procedures.

Pain frequently triggers fear. Even subconscious memory of pain can create fear. Fear can regress you to toddler status.

Sometimes you must get belly-to-belly with fear to resolve it. Rather than run and hide, face your fear. Look it in the eye and take its power. Fear dissolves in the Light of Truth. Bring Brazilian "attitude" to your Elephant Samba.

Samba derives from two African words. *Semba* refers to thrusting your navel while dancing. And, *samba* means prayer or adoration. Perhaps in this elephant dance, you adore and pray through the divine instrument of thrusting your navel! You confront and seduce your fear into submission.

The Elephant Samba activates your personal power. When you get face-to-face with fear and pain, a passionate new dance emerges. Think of it as a new form of prayer!

Soon in the dance, you will see that you can have fear or you can trust God. You can't have both. You must choose between fear and faith. It's that simple. Dancing the samba with a hefty-sized elephant demands trust in a Higher Power!

With the following dance steps, you can face any fear around needles, medical procedures, chemo, surgery, or pain. **Go belly-to-belly with fear and pain. Dance the Brazilian Elephant Samba! Ole!**

Gratitude Embrace

- To begin the dance, embrace your partner.
- Use gratitude to embrace the medical procedure, including its fear and pain. See the procedure as an ally bringing you to your goal of perfect health. See the fear and pain as opportunities to grow closer to God.
- The pain of the procedure is a small price to pay for the benefits of new life and health. Adore your dance partner.
- Healing begins with gratitude. Be grateful for doctors, nurses, hospitals, clinics, medical procedures, medicine, and needles.

Stay Present

- Fear lives in the past or the future. To avoid fear, stay in the present. If you stay present, fear diminishes.
- Use conscious breathing to stay in the Sacred Now. Count each inhale and exhale to stay focused. Repeat the cycle when you reach 10. Visualize each number in color.
- During crisis, relax. Consciously release stress—from the top of your head to the bottoms of your feet.
- Stop. Inhale. Exhale. Smile. Ground and center yourself. Remember God.
- Use your grounding skills to stay in your body. Think of your feet. Drop an anchor into the earth's core.
- Fear takes you up and out of your body. Being present in your body returns you to the Sacred Now and healing.
- You can't heal your body unless you are in it.
- Fear and pain decrease if you stay present.
- Feel the goodness of this moment. Notice the parts of your body that feel good. Magnify their vitality.

- Remember there is no heaven except what is here, now. There is nowhere to go, nothing to do. Receive heaven in this moment. Find richness in the now. The Sacred Now is your ally.
- The scared now is the Sacred Now—just move a letter. Shift your thinking from catastrophe to your Divine Self. Invite God into your now.

Ignore the Fear

- You have your life to live. You can spend it shrinking in fear. Or, you can ignore the fear and enjoy your life.
- Go Brazilian. Choose passionate enjoyment of life over fear. Let the dance move on. Look past your dance partner in arrogant disregard. Shake your bootay! Celebrate Rio de Janeiro and Carnival in the theater of your mind!
- Your mind can only think of one thing at a time. You can think of fear or something else. Choose something else!
- Treat fear like an annoying, naughty child who tries to grab your attention. If you ignore the intrusive child, he gives up and plays elsewhere. Ignore the fear. Place your attention on mantras, singing, clapping, TV, etc.
- Break the fear trance. Move your body. Change your location. Chair-dance to music. March around the room to Sousa music.
- "Feel the fear and do it anyway," as Susan Jeffers says in her book of the same title.
- Once when I was complaining about fear, my Mother said, "Most of the things I feared in life never came true. What I should have worried about never entered my mind!" Fear is not a reliable ally. Ignore it. Focus on the good things in your life!

Replace Fear with Faith

- To fight fear, replace negative with positive thoughts.
- Replace fear with faith. Martin Luther King said, "Faith is taking the first step even when you don't see the whole staircase."
- Trust God's loving plan for you. God's plan is always the highest, best, most glorious gift.

- Replace fear with fighters who will protect you. Call on Archangel Michael and his battalion of defender and protector angels. They will champion you and keep you safe.
- Remember the Wings of God. When you're afraid, run under God's Wings—like a baby bird running to it's mama. Feel the comfort, safety, and shelter.

Keep Your Eyes on the Prize

- Don't be fooled by apparent failure. It is temporary. Don't be defeated by "endless procedures." They will pass.
- Don't drain your power with negativity. Instead, keep your eyes on the prize. Rivet your eyes on victory, your complete healing.
- List the benefits you receive from your treatment.
- Go toward the prize, not away from the pain.

See Past the Procedure

- When fear of the procedure hounds you, meditate on how you will feel after it's finished. Anchor in the future.
- Prepare your bed for your return. Set a rose on your pillow. Place a friendly stuffed animal to greet you. Write a congratulatory note to yourself for completing another medical procedure. Feel how good it will be to snuggle into your cozy nest for a good night's sleep with the scary events in your past.
- Set a reward for yourself on completion, such as a candy bar, sitting in the sun, watching a video, calling a friend, buying a new outfit, or having a long luxurious bath.
- Go toward the reward, rather than away from the pain.
- Can you see beyond the medical procedure? Train yourself to see past the procedure to a vibrant future.

Strengthen Your Resolve

- There is no way out but through.
- Affirm your victory.

Blessings

- Before each medical procedure, repeat a blessing such as, "May this medical procedure go smoothly with minimum pain and maximum success." Visualize this. Feel it happening.
- Bless yourself frequently throughout the day! Say, "I am the perfect child of a loving God." "May the Light bring all that I need for comfort and healing." "May the blue sky wrap around me and keep me free."
- Night blessing: "May the night give back more than the day took away."

Angels

- Prior to a medical procedure, call upon your Angel Cradle. Lie back and feel the Angel Cradle draw close around you. Look up into the glorious eyes of your angels. Each angel has a different specialty to serve you. Learn each angel's name. Ask about her specialty. Angels of comfort, peace, detachment, trust, healing, strength, protection, renewal, and faith gather around you. Feel their arms and love supporting you. Enjoy the relaxing rhythm of swinging in your Angel Cradle.
- Send teams of Joy and Praise Angels ahead to prepare success in your procedure. See a carpet of sparkling gold Light unroll before every step in your new day.
- Visualize your Healing Angel Team in a circle surrounding you during the medical procedure. Feel their protective force-field of Divine Light keeping you safe. See angels above your doctors and nurses guiding them. Visualize the entire room protected by a Cocoon of Golden Angel Light. Feel joy and success in your bones as you rehearse the medical experience.
- Long ropes of Healing Blue Crystals suspend from the ceiling to the floor all around you. See them dazzling with God's healing blue Light and protection. You can reach out and touch them to steady yourself inwardly at any time. Use them to stabilize.

Needles and Medical Procedures

- Needles are your friends. They work for you. You hired them.
  They are here to help you. You pay for them. You are their
  boss. You are in control of them. Each one brings you closer to
  your goal of complete healing.

- To distract your attention from fear of needles during the
  procedure, ask the nurse about her life, her kids, and her travels.
  Write about it later in your journal. Remember the names and
  lives of medical personnel that you see frequently. Updating
  their stories is like watching a favorite TV series. It takes your
  mind off your troubles.

- Tell the nurse about your life. During bone marrow extractions,
  with my doctor's permission, I rambled on about some of my
  favorite memories. I especially enjoyed describing my daughter's
  Hawaiian wedding. The happy details distracted my mind from
  the painful medical procedure.

- At one point in my hospital stay, I was in an emergency where I
  was semicomatose. Eight nurses gathered around my bed to revive
  me. I had described my daughter's Hawaiian wedding to so many
  of them during previous difficult procedures that several shouted
  out, "Tell us about your daughter's wedding. What did the beach
  look like? Can you see the ocean? And the tiki torches?" My own
  self-healing technique came back to help me!

- Imagine that each medical procedure is a balloon in a room
  filled to the ceiling with balloons. To receive full healing, your
  job is to puncture all the balloons. Each needle you receive
  pierces a balloon and brings you closer to total health. Every
  needle advances your healing.

- Each medical procedure is a step toward your goal of complete
  healing.

- Small steps bring you to a great new place. Value even tiny steps
  forward. In the movie *Contact*, Ellie's father taught her to use a
  telescope to track celestial bodies. When she became impatient,
  he said, "Small steps, Ellie. Small steps." She later became a
  famous astrophysicist working in Project SETI, researching

extraterrestrial intelligence. Her initial small steps led to important scientific discoveries.

- As Lao Tzu says in *Tao Te Ching*, "The longest journey begins with a single step."

How Pain Works

- Pain contracts your field of attention. It can shrink your space so there is no room for you or your God connection.
- Don't confuse your identity with your pain. You are not your pain.
- Your True Identity is immense, infinite, eternal, and unchanging. Your Divine Source goes far beyond the pain. Remember who you are.
- Spirit expands your consciousness. It is an antidote to pain.
- When pain comes, ask the following questions: Who am I? Where is my power? Am I sourcing from God? Or false-sourcing from external events? What are the facts? What is the Truth? What is passing? What is permanent? What is ephemeral? What is eternal?
- Pain always passes.
- When pain comes, ask Why am I willing to endure this? What am I learning from the pain? What benefit will the pain bring? What is my reward?
- Keep your reward in mind continuously, night and day. It will expand your spirit.
- Go toward your reward, not away from the pain.

Construct Refuge with a Saint

- When pain comes, concentrate on Mother Mary, Jesus, Mohammed, Moses, Buddha, Lao Tzu, Krishna, or any of your favorite saints. The pain and the saint are happening simultaneously. Choose to concentrate on the saint.
- Your attention may wobble back and forth. Don't judge yourself. Keep returning to your saint.

- Be absorbed in the divine qualities of your saint. Feel the Godly presence. Describe the holy comfort. Receive love from your saint.
- Use your five senses to vitalize the connection with your holy helper. Hear his loving words. Feel his love. Give the love a fragrance. Associate your saint's love with a symbol, icon, or visual image. Find a taste that reminds you of your saint's energy. Feel your saint's touch. Watch your saint move.
- When the pain is great, let the angels take you away into Christ's Golden Love Embrace. Like a baby in his father's arms, feel yourself safe and secure in Christ's arms. He is a master of love and healing.

Divine Refuge

- "Established in the Void," Zen Buddhists call it. Be anchored in the silence of your own internal Godspring. Be solid and quiet. Feel apart from the events of your life. The immaculate, pure emptiness of the Void is a welcomed refuge when you are in pain.
- Find the part of you that is untouched by pain. Go there. This is your God Source.
- Find the part of you that has lived and died many times and is still unchanged. Go there. This is your God Source.
- Construct refuge in your God Source.
- Know the part of you that is one with God. Your God Self has access to infinite healing, intelligence, and supply.
- Your God made you and all that is. She can re-make you!
- To align with deep, profound peace and healing, memorize the Twenty-Third Psalm. Repeat it during medical procedures:

The Lord is my shepherd;
I shall not want.
He maketh me to lie down in green pastures.
He leadeth me beside the still waters.
He restoreth my Soul.
He leadeth me in the paths of righteousness
for his name's sake.

Yea, though I walk through the valley of the shadow
of death,
I will fear no evil.
For thou art with me.
Thy rod and thy staff shall comfort me.
Thou preparest a table in the presence of my enemies.
Thou annointest my head with oil.
My cup runneth over.

Surely, goodness and mercy shall follow me all the
days of my life.
And I shall dwell in the house of the Lord forever.

Your Victory Party

- When in pain, fast-forward to your Victory Party. Stand in Victory Day with all your friends and family celebrating your complete healing. Look back at today's challenge. See it as a link in a chain of events carrying you to victory.
- There is a path to your victory and perfect health. See the Healing Path. Others have walked it. So can you. Forget your doubts. See the Path zigzagging, vague, and fuzzy at first; then distinctly shining in Divine Light. See the end of the Healing Path with your welcoming Victory Team cheering you and your perfect healing.

Copy-Cat Healing

- Talk to the hurting cells in your body. Tell them to copy the happy, healthy cells in your body.
- Find the place in your body that is untouched by pain. Absorb its energy. Imitate it throughout the rest of your body. Multiply the good feeling until your whole body vibrates with healing.
- Tell the hurting cells to normalize by copying the billions of healthy people in the world.

- Fill your whole body-balloon with God's miraculous, natural, healing energy. Inhale healing into every part of your body.
- See the cells of your entire body made new. See them bright, healthy, and shining—like newly minted coins.

Surrender into God's Hands

- There are more important things in life and the universe than your personal plans and desires.
- God's in charge. Each day is his decision. You will leave the earth at the moment God has designed. No sooner. No later.
- God runs things while you're asleep! God doesn't make mistakes.
- The outcome of this medical event is already written in your Soul Contract. Relax and trust. The outcome is perfectly designed to help you reach your next step in growth.
- Surrender judgment. Accept your destiny. Remember, whatever happens could not be otherwise.
- Open your clenched fist. Place your burdens and suffering in God's loving hands. They are too heavy for you to carry. Let God carry them.
- Feel the hands of God supporting you—just as he holds the earth in space.
- Let go and let God support you.

Time/Space Machine

- Expand time. Fast forward 1,000 years in the future. Look back on today's pain. Notice how small it appears in the eternal river of time.
- Expand space. Go to the moon in your imagination. Notice how your perspective changes. See how insignificant your pain is in the infinite mosaic of cosmic evolution and the expanding universe.
- Expanded consciousness reframes your perspective. Go up your God Ladder. Wear your God Glasses. Time/space expansion helps you reassign meaning and value to your pain.

The Boston Elephant Ballet—Distract Your Mind from Pain

The glory is not in never failing, but in rising every time you
fail.
—Chinese Proverb

The Elephant Ballet is performed "sur la pointe." Fashioned after Walt Disney's *Fantasia*, the elephants are twirling, fat-legged, elegant, and self-satisfied in their glorious pink tutu skirts. The Ballet Elephant is a proper Bostonian. She walks with her trunk elevated.

Moving with utmost rotund grace, these skillful steppers glide past the pain. Hefting heavy body-cargo, they thrill to dramatic sweeps of motion. With leaps and arabesques, they teach you to keep moving in the pain dance. Overcome the weightiness of your situation.

Absorbed in other realms—perhaps chasing visions of their own pretty selves—the Ballet Elephants specialize in easy distraction from the "real world." These ballet behemoths are strongly established in fantasy. Some of them wear tee shirts saying, "I've given up my search for Truth. Now, I just want a good fantasy!"

In shiny, pink satin toe-shoes, Ballet Elephants chase invisible baubles. Like a baby's eyes tracking colored lights, these jumbos delight in life as a plaything. They pursue the slightest play-pretty giving them pleasure—whether color, taste, sound, fragrance, touch, or good emotions.

Let these smooth-stepping giants inspire you to glide past the pain. Trip the light fantastic in elephantine mimicry. Distract your mind with anything that delights or comforts you. Treasures are for YOU. Unashamedly indulge and exaggerate your distraction. Let pleasure hypnotize and transport you.

Use the **Boston Elephant Ballet to distract your mind from pain:**

Change the Channel of Your Mind

- Imagine a round TV channel-changer on your ear. When your mind fixates on pain, reach up and turn the dial.

- Use your Allies List to find a new station. Read your Prayer Team List. Look at pictures in your Prayer Team Album. Absorb their love and positive energy.
- Another distraction skill: Close your eyes and turn them up toward your third eye. This simple act can shift your attention from pain. Remember the gospel song, "When you look up, you can't feel down."
- Imagine you are in a soft, warm, comforting bath, surrounded by golden candlelight. Feel, see, hear, and know the relaxation of the bath. It is like a warm ocean wave, rocking you in the arms of God.

Magnify Gratitude and Beauty

- Gratitude and beauty are express elevators to God's heart. Use them to distract from pain.
- Count your blessings. Read Your Gratitude List. Prepare Your Daily Harvest Necklace. Remember Your Lifetime Treasure Box.
- Fixate on beauty. A wind-up music box with moving parts makes a perfect multi-sensory distraction. Use your willpower to enjoy even the slightest beauty.
- Merge with anything of beauty in the room. Unify with it. Bring it into your body. Take it's healing. Feel God loving you through the beauty.

Humor Heals

- Facing catastrophic illness, you must balance seriousness with humor. Humor is a health insurance policy. Throughout the day, practice joking with nurses, doctors, friends, and family.
- Norman Cousins healed himself of a life-threatening disease by watching *The Three Stooges* and comedy videos several hours each day. He used laughter as medicine.

- Watch *The Best of Saturday Night Live* videos according to either year or artist, such as Chris Rock, Phil Hartman, Dana Carvey, Mike Myers, Steve Martin, or Eddie Murphy.
- Enjoy comic concert videos by Jeff Foxworthy, Dennis Miller, Richard Allen, Paul Reiser, Billy Crystal, Robin Williams, Victor Borge, Johnny Carson, Whoopi Goldberg, Lily Tomlin, George Carlin, Phyllis Diller, or Dave Chappelle.
- Regularly view funny TV sit coms to shift your mood.
- Read joke books at night before bed and during depression.
- Check out the *Reader's Digest* humor sections.
- Explore Internet joke sites. Google *jokes.*
- Ask friends to e- or snail mail jokes to you.
- Listen to humorous audios by Swami Beyondananda and Garrison Keillor. Your spirits lift imagining Lake Wobegon "where the women are strong, all the men are good-looking, and all the children are above average."
- During medical procedures, ask a friend to read jokes to you. This really helps!
- Memorize good jokes to repeat during your alone times and with friends. This keeps your memory working and supports your healing.
- Cut cartoons from the daily newspaper.

Inspirational Reading

- Start each day with an inspirational keynote. Reference it frequently throughout the day. Choose from the following daily messages: the *Daily Word* published by Unity Village (Unity, Missouri), Louise Hay's tear-off calendar, the Anonymous Work's great books of inspiration *Courage to Change* and *One Day at a Time in Al-Anon*, Eileen Meyer's *The Road to Harmony: Day by Day*, Sarah Breathnach's *Simple Abundance.*
- Memorize positive slogans to strengthen your internal refuge and distract from pain.

- Savor morning devotional reading for 15 minutes. This is your time just for you. Align with God and charge your energy-battery for the day. Choose from the following:

    - Inspiring books such as the *Bible, Chicken Soup for the Survivor's Soul* by Canfield and Hansen, *Kitchen Table Wisdom* by Rachel Remen, *Tuesdays with Morrie* by Mitch Albom, *The Prophet* by Kahlil Gibran, *Hinds' Feet on High Places* or *Mountains of Spices* by Hannah Hurnard, *The Emmanuel Book* by Rodegast and Stanton, *The Holy Man* by Susan Trott, *Hope for the Flowers* by Trina Paulus, Deepak Chopra books, Thich Nhat Hanh books, *Making Miracles* by Paul Pearsall.
    - Poetry, especially Rumi and Hafiz.
    - Biographies of spiritual or historic leaders.
    - For more inspiration, see "Bibliography" at the end of *Elephants in Your Tent.*

- Read children's books, such as *The Little Engine that Could, The Little Prince,* and *The Velveteen Rabbit.*
- Ask others to read to you. Snuggle with a favorite blanket, the way you did as a child.
- If you are not up to reading, listen to inspiring talking tapes. See the "Audio Tapes" section at the end of this book for suggestions.
- Create your own inspirational audio tapes to hear when your spirit depletes. Tape-record favorite passages that give you strength.

Sing, Hum, Chant

- To oxygenate your blood, distract your mind, and renew your spirit, sing hymns. Easy access to mini-sermons, hymns provide a quick pick-me-up to elevate your mood. Absorb their positive energy.
- Internet sites offer words and music to sing along with. Do a Google search for hymns, rock 'n roll, country western, ballads, folk, or popular songs. Sing along as if you are a famous singing star.

- Trinity Broadcasting Network (TBN) on TV presents regular gospel singers.
- Practice toning. Fill the room with sound. Feel it vibrate in your body.
- Chant OM to align with God.
- Repeat mantras. Use mala beads to repeat chants. Repeat the Hail Mary using rosary beads to feed your Soul and distract your mind.

Listen to Beautiful Music

- Popular music can be inspiring, e.g., Neil Diamond's "Jonathan Livingston Seagull."
- New Age music can soothe your nerves, e.g., Aeoliah's "Angel Love," Robbie Gass's "Om Namaha Shivaya," Robert Slap's "Eternal Om," or Dean Evenson and Li Xiangting's "Tao of Healing."
- Classical music is full of healing sounds such as Debussy's peaceful La Mer, Rachmaninoff's passionate 2nd Piano Concerto, Beethoven's awesome 9th Symphony, Bach's elevating B Minor Mass, and Chopin's revitalizing waltzes, mazurkas, and 1st Polonaise.
- Make a song collection of your favorite sounds for your iPod. Listen when you are too exhausted to do anything else. Soak up the good energy.

Watch Videos

- See the list of films under "Recommended Resources" at the end of this book. Films provide a great mini-vacation from pain.

Use TV

- You can split your attention from pain by watching TV.
- Let your body go on automatic dealing with chronic pain, while your mind focuses on the TV. Use this distraction with

bathroom pains, insomnia, or any routine pain you experience daily. TV distraction is less effective with acute pain—though there are exceptions.

- Pain can create aversion to times of day or places in your home. Use TV to counterbalance the pain.
- You feel less isolated in the disease-worlds, when you connect with your tribe through TV. It helps you to normalize.
- I used TV to relearn the language. When you are really sick, sometimes you go extremely far away. When you return, you have to relearn the alphabet, numbers, how to read and write, how to listen, how to walk, how to talk. TV helped me relearn these skills. I listened to the language of the planet many hours. I studied the sounds and behaviors, the way a baby learns to speak by copying others.

Reach Out

- To distract your mind from pain, reach out to friends. Ask for help. In order for divine and human beings to respond, you must first ask.
- Call your Prayer Team. Don't be embarrassed. It is a sign of strength to know when to ask for help. Friends feel complimented when you reach out to them. Ask them to pray for you. Say, "I need your support right now."
- Research shows survivors feel connected to others. Call one friend each day. Just hearing a friendly voice takes your mind off pain. Stay connected. Write a love note to a friend.
- Studies prove that talking to others in a similar situation is healing. Join a support group of peers. You feel less alone when others validate your healing journey.
- Call upon your internal Soul Council. Ask them for help. Draw strength from their pictures.
- Call for prayer support. Unity in Unity Village, Missouri has a 24-hour prayer line. When I had given up hope, they prayed for me—not only that my pain lift, but also that I live a happy,

healthy life. Their prayers actually work! According to scientific studies, prayer power improves healing.

Speak Out

- Break the pain trance, by talking aloud to the empty room, as if someone were listening. Tell all your news, good and bad. Research reveals you can heal yourself emotionally by talking— even if no one actually hears!
- Write a daily journal. Tell it everything—both the good and bad news. Release your emotions into the writing. Studies demonstrate that recovery is faster and more complete among those who regularly write about their healing journey. You can talk into a tape recorder if you don't like to write.
- Collect stuffed animals. Talk to them about your day.
- Tell your troubles to a trusted counselor or friend.

Disconnect from Your Body

- Learn to consciously dissociate. With acute pain sieges, go out of your body.
- Know that you are not your body. Repeat the chant: I am not my body. I am that which is greater.
- Use your Observer Mouse to gain distance from the pain.
- Travel around the cosmos. Like the Little Prince, see earth from another planet.
- Visualize your "special magical place." Construct that place. See every detail. Use your five senses to experience being there.

Play Games

- Play cards to distract from pain and pass the time. Play solitaire in your pain ballet.
- Play board games such as Scrabble, chess, backgammon, Monopoly, or checkers.

- Color in your coloring book.

Glide Aside

- The pain is none of your business. Distract yourself from it. Use anything that works. Read a magazine, consciously breathe, talk to a nurse, count your relatives, count your fingers and toes!
- Use your power of choice to think of anything other than the pain. Fantasize shopping. List your favorite foods, music, or people. Tell yourself a joke.
- Change your field of attention.

The Texas Elephant Line-Dance—Work with Pain

Do what you can with what you have wherever you are.
—Theodore Roosevelt

Get your pain in line with this country-style promenade. Imagine you are leading a line-dance with your pain-elephant cooperating. You are in charge. Become the line-boss of your pain. Hear your voice issuing commands. Feel the pain respond.

Use the Texas Elephant Line-Dance when you want to work with the pain.

Spiritual Hound Dog

- Pain operates like a yellow caution light signaling you to pay attention.
- Often, it points to a wound in your belief system, so you can heal it.
- Is your pain physical, emotional, mental, or spiritual? Follow the pain like a spiritual hound dog hot on the trail to the gift of learning. Let the pain lead you to unresolved issues.
- One definition says, "Pain is resistance." What are you resisting?
- Often, we resist our good and our growth. What do you not want to see? What do you resist resolving in your life?

Clean the Slate

- When you've suffered too many invasive procedures and too much pain, you must regroup to face another day. Each night, wash away the day's challenges.
- Practice scientific forgetting.
- Visualize cleaning the slate. Don't bring yesterday's losses into tomorrow. Erase the blackboard of your mind.
- Turn the page. See a bright, fresh, clean page for the new day.
- Visualize magical Silver Scissors severing all psychic ties to yesterday's trauma.
- See Archangel Michael's Sword of Truth cutting you free from negative memories.
- Cast painful experiences out of your energy field with a giant exhale. Banish negative memories from your Inner Kingdom.
- Be merciful with yourself. Forgive yourself any self-judgment. God forgives you. God releases you from the past.
- Sail on to a bright new future—either in renewed health or in God's embrace on the other side of the veil.

Compartmentalize Your Life

- Compartmentalize your life into positive and negative memories. Put a firewall between yourself and yesterday's defeat.
- When pain comes, think of a positive department of your life, perhaps friends, family, hobbies, or nature. Go to a positive time and place in your life.
- Review your Lifetime Treasure Box.
- Create a list of your recent victories—regardless of how tiny they are. Post your Victories List on your bulletin board and on your bathroom mirror. Read your Victories List daily. Read it aloud.

Pain Passes

- Time is on your side. Remember the story of the ancient monarch who asked his aide to create a short sentence that applies to anything in life. The aide responded, "This too shall pass."

- The best thing about pain is that it always passes.
- Pain contracts your attention, so you might not see beyond the pain. Einstein said, "If you are sitting on a hot stove, a second can feel like eternity. When you look at a beautiful woman, it could last forever!"
- Recall a pain that once felt everlasting and that went away. Acknowledge your past triumphs over suffering.
- Your current pain will also pass. All there is in life is change.

Pain Jail Alert

- When you are down in the pain pit read this: *There is a better time coming. Tomorrow will be better. Remember how pain fooled you in the past when you thought it would never end? Pain always passes!*

Anchor in the Future

- Visualize a Golden Cable. Follow it to its end which is free from pain. Use willpower to anchor yourself in the better day, free from pain.
- Can you see past the pain?
- Send your anchor out to a positive future.

God's Perfect Pearl

- My adversity training creates the irritant necessary to form the perfect pearl.
- I am creating God's perfect pearl.
- The pain is my friend. It is helping me in ways that my mind can't understand.
- There are worse things in life than pain.

Altar of Deep Surrender

- The great Sufi poet Rumi demonstrated trust in Higher Power when he said, "Whoever brought me here will have to bring me home."

- If there is pain, it can only exist by God's will. You have the strength to endure it. Practice trusting God. Fall into God's loving embrace.
- See yourself dressed in a sacred robe, lying on the sparkling crystal Altar of Surrender. You are totally surrendered. The hand of God lifts you into heavenly realms. Feel the breeze on your cheeks as you move from earth's heaviness to the peaceful higher realms. Give your life to God.
- Remember Michael Angelo's Pieta at St. Peter's Basilica in Rome. Mary holds the dead body of Jesus in her lap. Her hands are uplifted, open, and surrendering. This is Mary's crucifixion. She offers her most precious possession—her beloved son—to God in sweet sacrifice. She totally surrenders to God's unfathomable will. Mary knows how to love, surrender, and trust God. She loves God enough to give him her greatest treasure, even in the midst of her greatest pain. To surrender, you must trust God as Mary did. Little did she know that her surrender was part of one of the greatest miracles in human history—the miracle of resurrected life.
- Be willing to give God your greatest treasure.
- Imagine the surrender of personal will for Jesus to enlist his spirit to the crucifixion. Now that's trust!

Transcend into God's Smile

- One gift of pain is transcension.
- Transcendence is on the other side of surrender. Transcendence lifts you beyond your earthly self to the larger perspective of your God Self.
- Transcendence brings you to God union. The transcendent place is God's smile.
- Surrender shows what you lose. Transcendence and God union are what you gain. Keep your eyes on the prize.
- Think how Jesus dealt with the pain of crucifixion. Imagine his thoughts as he was transcending pain. Feel his deep knowing.

He understood that he was not his body or emotions. He anchored in God Spirit.

Be God's Greatest Lover

- Have you shown God your love today? The poet says, "Love is not love that does not manifest."
- Among lovers, yesterday's love is not good enough.
- Is your love for God haphazard and occasional? Do you only send God love if good things happen? Do you only pray during hard times? Or, is your love focused, steady, and consecrated in a daily way regardless of events?
- Do you feel God loving you, despite negative external events?
- God's love often comes through beauty and gratitude. Beauty is everywhere! Gratitude is for everything!
- Don't waste, squander, spill, or block God's love.
- Open like a flower to the sun and receive God's love—even in the midst of turmoil. Feel the ecstasy and bliss of God's infinite love for you. How much love can you receive?
- Let God glorify you with his love. Feel the majesty that is God inside you, now.

Invite God In

- When you are in the hell pains, will to feel God's bliss. Open your heart. Say, "God, enter me now." On the inhale, fill yourself with God's love. Keep inviting God in. Say, "I want to hear your voice, feel your touch, see you, and know you, God. Please enter my being from head to toe. Now!"
- Practice receiving God's love. Open the doors and windows of your heart, mind, and spirit to receive God's love. Let God in!
- Talk to God all day. Ask for help.
- God's presence is strongest among the sick and wounded. God is needed there. Enjoy the presence of God in your healing journey.

- Move from thinking to feeling God in your body. Invite God in.
- Soften your heart. Healing begins with an open heart. You must open to receive.
- Fill your cup full of God's love. Feel God's love pressed down and spilling over into every area of your life.

Happiness

- Happiness is the ability to value and appreciate what you have. A student told the Indian sage Sri Nisargadatta, "I'm not happy with my life. I don't have . . . I want . . ." He gave a long list of his desires. Nisargadatta replied, "Turn it around. Be happy with what you have now. Forget the rest."
- Think about the things you can do, rather than what you can't do. Receive the good. Release the bad. As Sara Teasdale says, "Make the most of all that comes and the least of all that goes."
- Remember, it could be worse. There is always someone in a worse situation than yours.

Pain Transforms

- The function of pain is to transform.
- Pain is for a reason. It brings you nearer to God. Pain is a small price to pay for a great reward.
- During pain, use your Truth Compass: PERFECTION IS EVERYWHERE—ALWAYS. It transmutes negative to positive in your life.
- Emblazon this one basic Truth in your heart and mind. There will be times when you don't believe it. Discipline yourself to align with Truth. Find the perfection that is here, now.
- Find the wisdom gift in the pain. The great Lebanese poet, Kahlil Gibran, said, "Your joy of today is your suffering of yesterday, unmasked."
- Realize the pain is serving you. It is an ally.

- Guruji often said, "Through pain, you reach deeper into the well of infinite resource and manifest more greatness on earth."

Honor Your Pain

- Pain is one of your greatest teachers.
- Be gentle with your pain. Put space around it. Be merciful with yourself and your pain.
- As Thich Nhat Hanh says, "Don't run away from your suffering. Embrace it and let it reveal the way to peace."
- After major cancer surgery, Guruji said, "Pain teaches us to appreciate pain-free times. We know one from the other only by contrast. Behind the pain is a sweetness. God's loving guidance and care are always there. God is all we have to rely upon."
- Another time when asked about pain, Guruji said, "Hell resides inside Paradise. It is important to know Hell. Then you can expand your Paradise. Your Paradise must embrace your Hell."
- Pain forces you to expand your consciousness.
- Pain can be your liberator.

The Argentine Elephant Tango—Outsmart the Pain

Life is either a daring adventure or nothing.
—Helen Keller

To change,
A person must face the dragon of his appetites with another dragon,
the life-energy of the Soul.
—Jelaluddin Rumi

The tango is Argentina's national dance. There is passionate, predatory, caginess in the tango. Is this a dance of love or war? Talk about coexistence of the opposites!

Are the dancers one or two? He lurches one way. At the last fraction of a second, she joins him. She disappears down an imagined dark alley. He follows her. He flaps his wings to fly. A second later, she too becomes airborne.

There's no place one dance partner can go that the other doesn't follow, despite that suspense-filled moment of re-engagement. With the quick shift of a multiple personality, she changes directions, instantaneously becoming someone new. He magically meets her in a new world.

Dancing with pain, you too can become an expert tango dancer. Pretend you can match your partner's lightning-fast moves. Let skill follow fantasy. Use your South American bravado.

When pain dances fast and furious, match it move for move. Lurch, dip, and dodge. Become someone new—whoever you must become—to keep pace with the pain. Liberate the dancer inside you to follow wherever the pain leads.

All movement in the Argentine tango originates in the unity between the dancers. Bent knees and stiletto heels flash lightning-blade fast. There must be deep unity between partners—just to keep from maiming each other!

In your daily Elephant Tango, practice unifying with the pain. Think like the pain so you can move with it to protect yourself. Use your partner's body weight and momentum to your advantage, so you don't get crushed or stampeded.

Unless you understand your pain-partner's thinking, you can't out-smart it. Interview your pain. Develop a profile of its patterns. Use pain's information to your advantage in finding healing solutions.

Ironically, while tango bodies jet past in profound unity, the dancers' faces are detached—in high meditation. Contrasted with snapping bodies, the faces are aloof and immobile. The dancers' spirits are anchored in another realm.

Similarly, during your Elephant Tango, you must stay centered in your God Source. Keep part of yourself removed from the pain dance. Become the detached watcher even while you passionately dance.

Let nothing your pain partner does disturb your solid, inner core. In the midst of life-threatening emergencies, anchor your internal focus in God. Sustain your divine witness. Keep your spiritual distance, even during the intimacies of the dance.

You can stay in the dance without being trampled. Use the
Argentine Elephant Tango to outsmart your pain.

Pain Is War

- Be like a crafty general who understands his enemy's thinking.
  Study your pain's habits and patterns.
- Do certain people, places, or events trigger your pain? What
  time of day does it appear? What food activates it? What
  negative emotions or false beliefs accompany the pain? When
  did the pain originate? What does it want from you? What is
  the pain teaching you? What stops it?
- Assess your opponent. Develop a counter strategy to win the
  war.
- Use time between pain attacks to develop new strategies.
  Research on the Internet. Talk to others who have survived.
  Expand your information base through friends. Read about
  the latest discoveries related to healing disease.
- Enlist allies to help with your pain battle.
- Open new battle theaters. Use surprise tactics. Distract the
  enemy. Attack when you are strong. Choose your battles.
- Find solutions for a better life.

The Smart Runner

- Don't be trapped into thinking pain holds the only reality. Think
  beyond your current depletion.
- The smart runner may become exhausted early in the race.
  However, she remembers that her energy will renew later in
  the race. She says, "I will hunker down to get through the pain.
  I won't give my power to it. This pain will pass. New energy will
  come. I will not be tricked into thinking pain is my only reality.
  I will focus on the larger picture. I see the future when the pain
  disappears, my energy renews, and I win the race!"
- Can you see beyond your current situation?

Plant Your Flag in the Future

- Think to the other side of the difficult event. Plant your victory flag there.
- Fast-forward your life to the future, where you are happy and enjoying life. See yourself there.
- See past the pain.

Turn Pain to Your Advantage

- Like the t'ai chi warrior, turn your enemy's weight, momentum, and power to your advantage.
- Use the power of the pain to catapult yourself to God. Let pain be a call to prayer.
- When pain appears, train yourself with instant stimulus-response. Let the stimulus of the pain immediately trigger your God-trust in response. The second you feel pain, your trust in God shoots out blade-thrust-fast, with white-hot conviction.
- The more that is removed from your external life, the greater is the opportunity to construct internal refuge.
- Use every loss to create more space for God in your life.

Use Your Willpower

- Confront your pain. Tackle it! Don't be a victim.
- Like a war general, be resolute in your positive conviction for victory.
- Draw from infinite supply, intelligence, and healing. Anchor in your God Source.
- Fire up your willpower. Get on your horse and demand victory. Say, "In God's name, I claim what is mine! Healing is my birthright. My healing is manifesting now! So be it!"
- Shout, "Doubt and Fear, get out of my way! I'm coming through!" Replace them with an Army of Warrior Angels protecting and defending you.

A Mighty Healing Army

- Ask "How would the saints, Jesus, Moses, Mohammed, or members of the Planetary Hierarchy handle my situation?" Adopt their strategy. Enlist them to your Healing Army.
- You've heard of the Terminator. Archangel Gabriel is the Regenerator! He resurrects people from the grave. Put him on your Soul Council. Enlist his help daily.
- Saint Germaine is a member of Spiritual Hierarchy who specializes in transmutation and renewal. Known as the "Wonder Man of Europe" in the early 1700's, he looked the same for 100 years. He uses the violet ray of transmutation. The fleur-de-lis is his signature in meditation. He is a master of transmuting darkness to Light, negative to positive. Put him on your Soul Council. Call him to revitalize you. He will transmute the many negatives you encounter on the healing path.
- Immortal Master Babaji is the originator of Paramahansa Yogananda's spiritual lineage. Babaji is famous for his ability to manifest a completely new physical body. He is a master of regeneration. Call on him. He knows how to heal, restore, renew, and reconstruct you.
- The mighty healing power of the universal God comes to you through Archangel Raphael and his battalions of healing angels. Call Archangel Raphael to run his powerful green healing ray through every atom of your body and every aspect of your being. Open your heart. See, feel, hear, and know Archangel Raphael's green ray of healing in your body 24/7.
- The Lord Jesus, the Christ is a master of healing. He works with the gold ray of healing, forgiveness, and love. Work with him daily. He will teach you resurrection.
- Call these seniors in spirit to heal you. They will intercede with God on your behalf. They are powerful allies who can help you win your battle. They live to serve you.

Refuel with Pleasure

- Fighting pain is difficult work. Avoid pleasure deficit. Refuel with periodic pleasure throughout the day. Bring fresh supplies to the front lines of battle.
- Every 3 hours, give yourself a simple treat. Looking forward to a treat takes your mind off the pain. Look beyond the pain to your treat.
- Treats might include a walk, a phone call, a TV show, a video, a bath, a book, or a special food.
- Throughout the day, go toward the treat, not away from the pain.
- You'll be amazed how this tip refuels your will to live! Your pleasure treat restores the goodness of life.

Believe and Receive!

- There's always a way to success. Find the way! Ray Charles' mother told the blind singer as a child, "You might not be able to do things like a person who can see. But there are always two ways to do everything. You've just got to find the other way."
- Anything is possible! Open your thinking to receive your healing. Miracles abound throughout human history.
- Wake up! Don't fall asleep on the infinite intelligence, healing, and supply of your God Source. Claim the Truth of your being.
- Jesus said, "All things shall be done for one who asks."
- Ask and you shall receive.
- Command God to help you. Say to God, "You made me. Now, fix me!"

GOD MECHANICS

In God, there is always real life and eternal joy beyond passing
sufferings of the body.
—Swami Divyananda Saraswati

Journey to the Mind of God

Before enlightenment, the fish doesn't know it lives in water.
After enlightenment, the fish knows it lives in water.
—Judith Larkin Reno, Ph. D.

Has it ever occurred to you that you are seeking God with his eyes?
—Adyashanti, "Come to Your Senses"

You can never become what you already are!
—Karl Renz, *The Myth of Enlightenment*

I journey to the Mind of God frequently in my meditations. However, this time my Teachers want me to bring back conscious memory of the stations along the way—their names and functions.

I had been ill for five years. The doctors had found nothing, but I knew I was dying. Today's assignment was also to ask God if I would live or die.

To meditate was precious relief from thinking about survival. Meditation was a vacation from the pain. What luxury to relax my body and align with God. I felt protected, as my Guides led me through the many worlds to God's Inner Sanctum.

Traveling in my Light Body, I catapulted through outer space. Star clusters shot past me. White-hot balls of star-fire hurtled through supernova space. I honored the great star nurseries giving birth to baby stars as I passed. Jockeying through radiant star canyons, I marveled at frozen nebulae hanging suspended inside orange-purple, cotton candy fuzz.

I loved the quiet zones. The space between the stars was immaculate, pure, empty. It was comforting and familiar. I enjoyed going Home.

Moving at unearthly speeds, I tracked along golden rays that unfurled like royal carpet leading to my first stop, the Great Golden Sun. The Golden Sun was a powerful, loving Teacher. Its early spiritual initiations taught me, along with other spiritual trainees, to penetrate the Psychic Barrier between earth's reality and higher realms of consciousness.

Crossing the Psychic Barrier opened the candy jar of divine realms. They thrilled me after earth's pedestrian tedium. I remember the Golden Sun saying, "Now, you are free of earth's prison of time and space. You can move beyond limited locality. Enjoy the freedom and infinite intelligence of your non-local identity." How crude earthly realities seemed after romping in limitless realms!

Reliving past lives, lucid dreaming, time-tripping, bi-locating, seeing auras, radiatory healing—all came naturally, with the help of the Great Golden Sun. "Miracles are your birthright," the Golden Sun often said.

I especially loved the dream trainings. Time-tripping to past, parallel, and future lives, I gathered a treasure trove of spiritual insight and wisdom. I healed hundreds of past lives—both my own and other people's.

Walking through walls, breathing under water, and moving the clock-hands were basic exercises in lucid dreaming. I decoded and transmuted dreams while I was having them. I learned to expand and contract time.

Like a child playing with building blocks, I practiced my power to create—constructing and deconstructing dream worlds. Realities are fluid and plastic. You can re-shape them like play dough. The dream worlds unlocked my power to create in the waking dream of earthly life.

In early initiations, the Great Golden Sun filled me with ecstasy and deep love for God. It fueled me to pass tests in love, service, sacrifice, discipline, and right use of spiritual power. I studied leadership and followship. Profound surrender to my wise, all-loving, beloved God became daily fare.

Approaching the Great Golden Sun, I recalled the wonderful allies it had given me through the years. Each ally advanced my spiritual growth. My allies included angels, Planetary Hierarchy, deities from the many pantheons (Greek, Roman, Egyptian, Hindu, Christian, Buddhist, American Indian), spiritual guides, Intergalactic Brotherhood, power animals, nature elementals, and nature devas.

The allies taught me discernment and right action in the many realms. Under their tutelage, my identity dissolved and reinvented rapidly. With each reinvention, there was slightly less of "me" and more of God.

As spiritual initiations progressed, the Golden Light taught me to heal planetary karma and become a Planetary Server. Following the learning curriculum, I became a Light Worker and ultimately a Light Bearer transferring Light to others.

I traveled around the planet with teams of dedicated Light Workers installing the Planetary Light Grid for the New Wisdom Age. This important implant in the earth's energy body will last for the next two thousand years. It lays the foundation for many glorious, future growth-cycles as we enter the Aquarian Age.

Humanity is in the midst of planetary spiritual initiation. This is a time of grassroots enlightenment. Millions of Light Workers carry the same energy that Jesus did two thousand years ago. After doing miracles of healing, transmuting water to wine, multiplying loaves of bread, raising the dead, and walking on water, Jesus said, "You shall do these things and more."

Today, Light Workers around the world are blossoming just as Jesus predicted. Spiritually, it is an exhilarating time to be alive. Miracles abound. People are awakening to the mystical worlds at an unprecedented, accelerated rate.

Under the influence of the Golden Sun, I found my place on earth as a counselor and spiritual teacher. The Golden Sun's training involved many challenges, sufferings, victories, and miracles. It was never dull.

The Golden Sun is the Light of the Soul, the Divine Mother. She is non-judgmental, nurturing, and unconditionally loving. She interfaces earthly and divine realms, mediating between them. Each spiritual seeker must unify with the Golden Light and embody it in his auric field on earth.

I had first seen the Golden Light of my Soul in mirror meditations. I gazed in the mirror with a diffused and unmoving focus, looking at my third eye. Eventually, my face and body grew hazy. A two-inch outline of radiant white light emerged around my body. That was my etheric, energy body.

If I gazed long enough, I noticed colors radiating through my etheric envelope. Shaped like clouds and occasional symbols, the colors moved throughout my overall energy field.

Green in my aura meant healing for me. Blue was spiritual calmness. Red could be vitality or anger. Orange meant courage. Pink was love. Violet was Saint Germaine's transmutative ray helping me to clean up my act, transforming negative to positive energy. The Golden Light was the wise teaching presence of my loving Soul.

Though the journey was familiar, approaching major stations to God I felt like a supersonic jet passing through the sound barrier. My "hull" shuddered with almost unbearable, intensified power, straining every fiber to stay on course.

As I entered the kingdom of the Great Golden Sun, old forms dissolved. Like Basho's frog, in the famous Japanese haiku, I dove into a new world—rupturing earthly realities.

> Old pond
> Frog jump in
> Water crash!

I relished re-uniting with my old friend and beloved Teacher. Like a joyful, teenage dolphin, I frolicked in a sea of love. I dove exuberantly, bobbing and looping in the Golden Soul-Light.

Merging with the Golden Sun, I knew—as Basho had said— neither I, nor the Sun would ever be the same. The Golden Sun was reconstructed by me, just as I was redesigned by our blending. We informed each other in our union.

"Know yourself as God," my Soul often said. "You and I are one. We just manifest in different forms—or lack of it in my case! One is not better than the other. We are equal. It insults me when you denigrate yourself. Think of yourself as part of me and vice versa. You must expand your identity to contain both of us."

During this visit, my Soul infused me with love, compassion, joy, and beauty. My original team of spiritual teachers, the Wise and the Strong, greeted my return. It was wonderful to hear their Pure Voiced Teachings again.

After due time in this glorious immersion, my journey to the Mind of God resumed. With sweet good byes, I returned to my invisible cosmic track—once again catapulting through space.

I was now deep inside the Kingdom of Light. Colors nourished me like food. Rays of tart apple green, lemon yellow, and sweet peach reached though black, cosmic night—their laser fingers yearning to connect with a target.

The rays of sacred Light blessed me with their healing energies. However, I could easily sidetrack into their glorious worlds. Their temptations felt like the Sirens seducing sailors off course in Odysseus's heroic journey. The sailors were tied to the mast to avoid abandoning ship.

Without benefit of mast, I riveted my concentration on the Great Silver Sun, my next gateway to God. As I sped forward, the Golden Sun grew small and distant, until there was no longer a trace of it. I began traveling on a beam of radiant Silver Light.

The Silver Sun embodies the father principle of protection, detachment, and strength. Holding the power of Universal Law, the Silver Sun's unspoken message is "Don't mess with me." It is impossible to lie in its presence. The Light is so clear, there is nowhere to hide. This is the land of integrity, Truth-telling, and crystal clarity.

Merging with the Silver Sun, I recognized it as my own personal God Self. It links my Soul with the awesome, impersonal God Source—the Void. At each level of the journey Home, more of "me" dissolved.

I dropped layer after layer of personal self, as the impersonal vibration increased.

With the Silver Sun, I moved beyond subject/object duality. With my Soul, I had witnessed the experiencer of my life. I saw Judith living her life. At the Silver Sun, I lost even the witness level of selfhood. My God Self took me beyond duality into unitive consciousness.

In the Silver Light, every moment of my earthly existence replayed before me. This Grand Review usually comes at death. Watching the panorama of my life, I realized everyone I had ever mistreated was myself. I saw with immaculate clarity both my good points and my limitations. I saw my ignorance and my heroic courage.

The Silver Sun taught me to forgive my earthly self with deepest love, compassion, and mercy. I learned to forgive others, life—and even God. Until then, I hadn't realized how much I blamed God for the challenges in my life.

The Silver Sun wields the Sword of Truth. In the Clear Silver Light, I saw that my God concept was my own projection—my human invention. It was a composite of all that I had read, heard, seen, and experienced. I had constructed my personal God mainly from preconscious experiences of my mom and dad.

My ego's involvement in my God concept shocked me. Instead of clearly perceiving God, I merely invented God. Spiritually embarrassed, I felt denuded. The Naked Light stripped me of my old, out-worn God relationship.

More shocks ensued. In the Clear Light of Truth, I also had to admit my codependence with God. Codependence is giving to get. It is a form of manipulation, based on illusion and unworthiness.

Subconsciously, I believed that if I were a good girl, God would love me more. I would get more rewards—better health, more money, more love, etc. In effect, I was codependently earning God's love, rather than trusting and deserving it. I was dancing faster to please a lollipop God!

Once I saw my "disease to please," I realized I was unconsciously trying to control God through my "goodness." My Guides pointed out that spiritual codependence is common among today's spiritual initiates. However, their observation was small comfort!

Instead of trusting God, I had created myself as a false god with my assessments of good and bad. My earthly mind continuously chattered about how life **should** be—as if I had the one right way. Attacking God with my judgments, I made God wrong.

Imagine judging God! I examined my personal will run riot. There was no room for God's will in my Inner Kingdom. I was too busy telling God about his mistakes! Creating myself over God had to be the ultimate grandiosity!

As my Guide said, "You can have God or your human judgments. You can't have both!"

By definition, God is inscrutable. It is literally impossible to understand God. The human mind is of no use in the God realm beyond mind. How could I judge God? It was impossible.

Acknowledging my own ignorance, I began surrendering into the Great Unknowing. Gradually, I created space for the Great Mystery. My God grew larger and greater, beyond anything I could imagine.

The clear Light of Truth was not easy. Standing in its Ruthless Radiance was a grueling, though valuable rigor. The Silver Sun comforted me, "Remember, enlightenment is grieving the loss of many illusions."

The Silver Sun did not entirely bereave me of my personal God. Since God is both immanent and transcendent, personal and impersonal, there is a genuine, legitimate human need for a personal God.

The Silver Sun said, "Your personal God Self is essential to your wholeness while you are human. You need a safe, human bridge to the vast, impersonal, universal God Source—the Void. You think I'm fierce, just wait until you dissolve in the infinite Cosmic Void!"

The Silver Sun continued its deconstruction—alias demolition—service. It revealed more illusions in my understanding of God. My humanly invented God was a tyrannical, uncompromising, hard taskmaster. I had blamed God for all the pain, suffering, and injustice in the world. At a deep level, I had been at war with God all my life.

One definition of enlightenment is "To take back all your projections." I had a lot of work ahead, undoing the blame and false beliefs I had heaped on my personal God.

Trusting God's will beyond my own wouldn't be easy. The only way I could surrender was if I had a truly trustworthy, benevolent God, rather than my old punishing God. I quickly realized I had to reinvent my God!

In the magical Light of the Silver Sun, the Land of Truth, I momentarily saw through God's eyes. The veil of human ignorance lifted. I saw that humans learn through pain.

We come to earth to receive its resistance. Earth's intense duality—hot/cold, male/female, good/bad, up/down, pleasure/pain—is not available other places in the universe. The resistance of pain is an essential teacher for humans.

Pushing against daily duality, we create friction, a spark of awareness, and eventually the Light of consciousness. Burning through ignorance, we burn off karma. Through earthly pain, we discover our divine side.

I saw that God gave me the exact pain I needed to fulfill my Soul Contract. Through pain, I awakened, transcended, and dissolved past karma. I became new. The pain re-created me. It sacralized me. It purified my false beliefs and made me whole.

Inside pain was the gift of growth. God was never punishing me. Like all humans, I needed certain, precise suffering to learn particular wisdom assignments.

The pain wasn't about me. It wasn't personal. I hadn't done anything wrong. Pain is just the way humans learn on earth.

My Guides pointed to the service my suffering provided for humanity. The transmutation I provided went far beyond my human ability to comprehend. All of it was God's creation, having little to do with "me." I was just God's instrument. And, I had thought I was in charge!

From the vantage point of the Silver Sun, I saw the divine plan. I realized how lucky I had been. God had consistently loved and protected me. Through all my incarnations, I had never died. Now, I could harvest the wisdom and love from the suffering times.

The intense Light of Truth in the Silver Sun reveals all error thinking. If God had an eyeball, the Great Silver Sun was it! No part of me went unexamined. I knew that eventually I would cycle through the Silver Sun and return immaculately pure and empty to the next leg of my journey Home.

Contrasting with the loving embrace of the Golden Sun, the Silver Sun was severe. However, after the initial shock of realizing the Sword of Truth was whittling "me" away, I relaxed and enjoyed lightening up. The intense, Silver Radiance gloriously deconstructed me. It was a veritable weight-loss chamber!

The personal God Self specializes in advanced lessons involving identity, non-attachment, purification, surrender, crucifixion, forgiveness, transcension, and God union. Every atom of the spiritual initiate's body changes to contain the elevated Silver vibration of the personal God Self. The initiate must embody its electric silver-white radiance.

The Silver Sun's training can involve thousands of incarnations. However, earth's vibration is currently accelerating. So, spiritual students may learn in a few months what once took an entire incarnation. These are indeed privileged times to hold a position on earth.

The Silver Sun attuned me to the impersonal life. I appreciated its gifts of cosmic perspective, emotional sobriety, and refuge in immaculate peace. I discovered new reverence for pure emptiness, silence, non-doing, and space.

In addition, the Silver Sun taught me that I am both everything and nothing. Though paradoxical, both teachings are true.

The Golden Sun had given me the bells and whistles of the siddhis—the magic powers that eventually come to many spiritual initiates. The Silver Sun took them away as too heavy a burden to carry in the nakedness of returning to God.

Again, I faced the paradox of accretion and renunciation. Both paths lead to God. Both are necessary spiritual teachings. Two spiritual paths, labeled "More" and "Less," arrive at the top of the same holy mountain!

Purified by the Cosmic Sauna, I emerged from the Silver Sun to resume my journey Home to the Mind of God. I entered a zone that always stunned me.

Thus far on the journey, I was occupied visually—first by the Golden Sun of my Soul, then by the Silver Sun of my personal God Self. The initial phase of the quest was about Light.

Now, as if my eyes were plucked from my head, I could see nothing. Disoriented, I didn't even know which end was up. I flipped and spun, searching for the familiar energy-track to the Mind of God. Exhausted, I surrendered and floated upside down.

Slowly adapting to the new medium, I heard the Inner Voice say, "Congratulations. You have deconstructed enough to enter the God Sound." No longer led by Light, the God Sound became my guide.

The God Sound is the sacred voice of the universe. Some call it the music of the spheres. It is an ethereal vibration informing matter of its divine origin. All manifest form dances to its tune. You can hear the God Sound in nature. Behind the busy cacophony of birds and insects is a high-pitched sound—fine as spider's silk—that drills deep inside your brain.

The God Sound integrates your brain hemispheres. During meditation, it eases you into a transcendent state, beyond your body. The God Sound is the threshold to God's Inner Sanctum.

The God Sound is always with you. It is the still, small sound behind everything else. You may miss it, because it is so close. It is difficult to discern a background sound that never stops. Just as the fish doesn't know it is in water, the God Sound is such a part of you, you may not recognize it at first.

To be so close to the raw sound of God was enchanting. I felt like a baby lulled in its mother's womb, listening to the steady rhythm of her heartbeat; comforted by the white sound of her rushing blood and body fluids. The baby knows no separation from her mother.

Similarly, I felt no separation from God, except a thin shard of awareness—the way you feel when you're falling asleep. A comforting security blanket, the God Sound confirmed my profoundly intimate relationship with the universal God.

The God Sound is the last familiar landmark for the mind. Humans traffic heavily in the life of the mind. Personal identity is an invention of the mind. It is quite a trust walk to transcend the mind and its many investments. I knew the God Sound's job was to move me into the Void.

The Sacred Sound is the thread of continuity running among the many realms of consciousness. The Hindus chant Om to find this last stop before the Void. Though it is a crude tool contrasted with the ethereal God Sound, Om can align you with God Source.

The God Sound is the zone between Light and the Void. It is the lip of God—God's voice, as it were. It is the sound of God Spirit.

Hearing is the last sense to go when you leave the human experience at death. It is also the first sense to arrive as the zygote develops into a fetus.

My Inner Guides reminded me, "Death and sleep are the same journey that you are now traveling. It is a natural, familiar journey—though most humans forget it.

"Every night, humans pass through the gateways of the Golden and Silver Suns. Next, they move into the Sound Current. Finally, they dissolve into the Void, merging with impersonal, universal God Source for retooling and renewal.

"Indeed, many times in an instant throughout both day and night, each human dissolves into the Godspring and emerges out of it. At speeds faster than the eye can see, humans literally pulsate—flashing on and off. They continuously manifest and unmanifest—deconstructing into the Void and reconstructing on earth.

"The censoring mechanism of the brain blocks memory of the journey Home so humans can focus inside earthly reality. Without training, it could be disconcerting to disconnect from earthly time/space and experience the infinite, eternal Void. Cosmic whiplash is a hazard!"

My Teachers had often explained how the brain is a reductive agent. It mercifully filters the many cosmic realities and time/space corridors. Brain-blocking concentrates the mind on a particular earth-life assignment.

Most humans could not tolerate too many out-of-body experiences. Past-life memories could prematurely explode their earthly reality and human identity. Without the safety net of metaphysical training, they could not integrate cosmic information. They could get spiritual digestion—mega-big time!

My Teachers continued imparting valuable information. "Someday there will be a camera filming human consciousness looping up and down the God Ladder—from spirit into matter and back again. The camera will show your cosmic blipping off and on each second. It will show 'you' dissolving in the Void."

Eeek!!! Standing on God's lip, I was literally about to be swallowed by the Void. Despite their good intentions, my Guides weren't helping. Their description was not much of an incentive—let alone a travel promotional!

I clung to God's lip. At least the God Sound provided some structure, regardless of how slight.

Trying to pump me up for the Big Leap, my Guides continued, "You've done this journey innumerable times. There **is** a return loop. There is no way the Real You can die! When will you trust that? You confuse your body with your identity!"

The Guides showed me the reverse ride down the God Ladder from the Mind of God into matter, back into my body. They said, "Someday, the cosmic camera will make it easier. If you see the ride, both up and down the God Ladder, you will feel safer. Each ride up and down the Ladder reconstructs and renews you.

"On the ride down the Ladder, the camera will show the idea that is 'you' emerging from God's Mind. You gather vibratory power moving through God's lips. The God Sound motorizes your trip from idea into matter.

"Spirit first manifests as sound. The God Sound holds the secret of manifestation. The *Bible* says, 'In the beginning was the word. The word was made manifest.' All manifest form emerges from the God Sound. Truly, your word is your power to create.

"The entire Hindu Vedantic tradition rests on the sacred power of sound to create. The original Sanskrit alphabet captures the essence of each earthly object in its naming.

"Fortified with sound, God's concept continues the journey down the Ladder into matter. 'You' move from the Mind of God (the Fertile

Void), to God's lips (God Sound), through his eyes (Light), and then into your physical body.

"Earthly form is gravity-entrapped Light. Light and Sound are primary agents of manifestation. They help to create earthly life.

"On the cosmic assembly line, as you enter Light realms, you receive your God Self which enlivens God's blueprint, formatting 'you.' A wise father, your God Self is your God-link, guiding you. Like the Tin Man in the *Wizard of Oz*, you also receive a heart. A loving mother, your Soul nurtures you.

"Next, our probable human enters earth's gravitational field. 'You' finally emerge into physical realms.

"You see, the journey up and down the God Ladder is normal and natural. You have done it countless times. The only difference now is that you are conscious of the journey Home. Each ride regenerates you."

The Teachers' discourse regarding the return ride comforted me. I was ready to drop the last vestiges of humanness and merge with my God Source. I made friends with the great Void.

I told myself, "After all, physical construction is just a local custom. It's a provincial habit I learned on planet earth. The Void is the more natural state. The Sacred Void is universal, not just a regional convention."

I surveyed the vast unconstructed Matrix, full of all potential, out of which all manifest form emerges. The Void is God's primary residence.

My Guides often spoke of its universal presence. "The Void is everywhere, always. You are never separate from it. It neither comes nor goes. It is in all that is.

"Imagine taking a magical tour inside an atom, searching for solid matter. You soon discover the 'solid matter' is the size of a grain of salt relative to the Houston Astrodome. Ninety-nine percent plus of the atom is empty space—the Void! The atom is the building block of matter.

"If you journey further inside the grain of salt of 'solid matter,' you discover it is not solid. Rather, it is comprised of light.

"Continuing your journey inside the light, you discover it is continuously blinking off and on. 'Solid matter' is a strobe light, continuously dissolving into the Void and emerging out of it as it moves up and down the God Ladder. In continuous flux, the world of form is an insubstantial light show!

"Since the Void is omnipresent—in both matter and emptiness—it has knowledge of all that is. The Void is therefore omniscient. As the philosopher said, 'Knowledge is power.' Being omniscient, the Void has power over all. Thus, the Void is omnipotent.

"Omnipresence, omniscience, and omnipotence are the three qualities of the universal God Source. The Void is the immanent, universal, and transcendent Mind of God."

The moment I lept into the Void, I would merge with God. The magnetic attraction to my own Godspring was inevitable. The return Home was hard-wired into my design.

However, my human consciousness was leaping into a burning volcano—the throbbing chaos of deconstructed reality. My human side felt the terror of impending extinction. Talk about counter-intuitive moves!

As I leapt into the great Void, I abandoned any remaining personal identity. The human mind is of no value in this realm beyond reason. The mind is only a useful tool to reach the threshold of the Void. You use your mind to transcend the mind into spirit.

Trying to describe the indescribable Mind of God is folly at best. Universal God Source is so essential—so reduced—it is beyond form and concepts. Technically, there is no way to conceive of the Cosmic Void.

However, the human mind needs the comfort of a map of consciousness. I can describe the Mind of God as pure energy, infinite potential, and dynamic peace. Paul describes it in the *Bible* as the "peace that passes understanding."

A great warehouse of essences, the Void contains the building blocks of all form in the multiverse. The essences are the bricks, so to speak, before they become structure. Imagine merging with this energizing Cosmic Soup—full of all potential.

Don Juan, the spiritual teacher in Carlos Castaneda's books, once described psychically watching his friend die. His description matches my journey to the Mind of God.

As if in time-lapse photography, first his friend's body melted, returning into the earth. Then, one by one, the patterned elements of his emotions, mind, beliefs, personality, intuition, Soul, and spirit dissolved. Don Juan watched his friend evaporate!

The elements comprising his identity were demagnetized, no longer focused in their earthly format. With the liberation of death, they flew like homing pigeons back to their origin in the Godspring.

Death is the Great Unspooling. All that earth has woven deconstructs and returns to God Source for reassignment. This ultimate spiritual undressing relieves you of the heavy burden of earthly illusions. You return to the Fertile Void for retooling, renewal, and rebirth.

The Fertile Void is alive with potential, ready for use in the next creation that emanates from God's Mind—your next revision.

Though the Sacred Void is unconstructed, there is an intelligence or presence there. At first, it is almost indistinguishable. Imagine a magical room that is completely dark inside. There is a giant flywheel spinning at such a rapid speed that you can't see or hear it. However, you feel its presence when you enter the darkness. Similarly, you feel the awesome presence of God, once you acclimatize to the Void.

As I adapted to the Unconstructed Place, I experienced God rushing to meet me, as if she had been unutterably bored and desperate to see me. God was hungering for company in general. But, she was overjoyed to see me specifically. This welcome would be the same for anyone.

God was eager for my earthly information. She wanted to know how the human experiment was going, how the "device" she invented was working.

I was amazed to realize that God was as eager to see me, as I was to see her. God had the same passionate love to be reunited. She needed me as much as I needed her!

We were long-lost buddies, both talking at once, updating each other on our adventures. It was quite a gab fest! I downloaded my information about earthly experience into the Mind of God. And, God imprinted eternal principle and renewal in me. It was a balanced, fruitful exchange.

Our reunion reminded me of Rumi's poem describing a mouse and frog who meet every morning in the hollow of a riverbank. Stories instantly spill out of them as they open their hearts to each other. They easily share dreams and secrets, without fear. As Rumi says, "There's no blocking the speechflow-river-running-all-carrying momentum that true intimacy is."

From the perspective of the Mind of God, I immediately realized my questions about life and death were moot. It didn't matter whether my physical body lived or died since my human identity was ephemeral, like the mist. It was a vaporous light show—fabulous entertainment, but insubstantial.

Earth's light show was God's home entertainment center. "I" was one of God's TV/movie inventions. The fears, joys, triumphs, and failures, all made fabulous film. It was all play—God's wonderful *lila*.

I had come to the Mind of God to ask if I would live or die. From my unlimited God level, the question sounded like a joke. How could I die when I was eternal? How could I die when I was already dead! There is no life or death, just the endless strobe light of dissolving into and emerging out of the Void.

The endless strobe light has a hypnotic rhythm. Within its reality, there is no good/bad duality. There is dissolve-emerge and dissolve-emerge, in a beautiful, pulsating cosmic light show.

Life/death, pleasure/pain, all were dramatic conventions from a faraway place. Among cosmic travel destinations, earthly life is an exotic backwater. It is fascinating, but hardly conclusive or definitive. Earth was becoming a distant memory for me.

Once I got this far in my conversation with God, the two of us burst out laughing. Everything seemed hilarious. What was all that life and death struggle about on earth? What part of me hooked into believing the light show had substance? Why did I believe I had to fight to live? Battle against pain? Ha! It was all a cosmic joke.

I can still hear our laughter rolling down the cosmic corridors of infinite time and space as God and I discussed whether I would live or die. What ecstasy to laugh and be free! "I" was already dead. "I" had never lived! How do you carry on a discussion that doesn't exist? It was the best discussion I never had!

After my visit, I traveled the reverse journey from the Void of God Source, to the God Sound, into the Truth of the Silver Sun, back to the loving Golden Sun, then into gravity-entrapped form on earth. Once back on earth, it no longer mattered whether I lived or died. It all was perfect. What a great game! I was no longer trapped inside the game. I was free to enjoy it, both as a participant and an observer.

As earthlings, we are continuously on a journey Home. In my role as spiritual cartographer, I hope this map of my journey helps with your travels.

Drawing up the travel brochure and over-viewing the itinerary, I notice God's Laugh is the ultimate landmark!

Established in the Void

> *Is the butterfly dreaming he is a man? Or is the man*
> *dreaming he is a butterfly? This is enlightenment.*
> —Chuang Tzu, Taoist Master

After my journey to the Mind of God, I realized that God union had always been inside me. When I was in the Mind of God, I experienced complete union. There was nowhere to go, nothing to do. No life. No death. No good or bad. No difference. Only pure, open, rich peace.

After my journey, I took a distant overview of my personal life. I didn't take myself so seriously. I experienced healthy uncaring without the old urgency. I disengaged from my human drama.

I realized I had been codependent with my life—mistaking my life for my identity. I mistook the events of my life for my value. False-sourcing from people and events, I had invested my life with false meaning.

Returning to earth, I no longer allowed people or events to define me. Rather, I surrendered my life into God's care. I had found my true God Source.

"Be established in the Void," the Zen Buddhists advise. All my adult spiritual life I asked, "How do I anchor myself in nothingness? How do I build a firm foundation on nothing!"

Yet, my Spiritual Teachers continually repeated, "Anchor yourself in the Void." It was a frustrating koan.

After visiting the Mind of God, I found security in the Void. It is a relief not to carry the burdens of human life. I no longer "play God." I let God do her job.

Cosmic Blinking

Enlightenment is not awake, not asleep.
—Buddhist

The journey to the Mind of God and back to earth has two dynamics, yin and yang. Yin is extreme expansion, moving into spirit. Yang is extreme contraction, moving into matter.

In the ride up the God Ladder, matter evolves into spirit. In the ride down the God Ladder, spirit infuses into matter. Each ride up the God Ladder is an opportunity for renewal.

There is a relaxing strobe light effect as Light and the Void alternate. God inhales and exhales, constructing and deconstructing matter. Spirit and matter rhythmically commingle and separate, dissolving back into the Void.

In the Mind of God, I felt like a spark of light absorbed into darkness. "Gate. Gate. Paragate," is the ancient Sanskrit description of nirvana or God union. "Go beyond. Go beyond. Go beyond into extinction," is a translation.

The Buddhist definition of nirvana is "extinguished," as in extinguishing a flame when you blow out a candle. All sense of personal self extinguishes in God union. This unitive absorption— beyond duality—is the experience of God.

We continuously blink on and off, many times in a second, as we dissolve into the Void and emerge out it. We are all God blinking! To be a cosmic blink isn't so bad. Once you get used to it!

REINVENT YOUR GOD

Design a God

*At each new level of healing, in order to survive, I had to
reinvent my God. At first, I didn't realize God concepts
become obsolete as you cycle-up in growth.*
—Judith Larkin Reno, Ph. D.

In the healing journey, I often find my behavior, emotions, and the events of my life don't match my credo or my God concept. My idea of how I think it should be often doesn't match events.

Incongruity is a signal that I'm out of God alignment. To maintain structural integrity, I need a spiritual chiropractic adjustment!

Healing is wholeness. It takes vigilance to maintain structural integrity over all 7 levels of your being: physical, emotional, mental, intuitional, Soul, personal God Self, and impersonal God Source.

God is your chief ally in fighting pain and disease. It serves you to have clarity regarding who/what your God is. Your God relationship and concepts are essential to your healing.

As you advance in healing, you may experience a surprisingly new God and a new relationship with God. You may reinvent your God. Abandoning old cherished assumptions and beliefs, you may move to a new neighborhood in consciousness to find God.

The following section helps you become aware of your God concepts and relationship. God is a very individual experience. Everyone has a different God.

Your perception of God changes throughout a lifetime—according to developmental stages and needs. Before seven years old, most children are not particularly concerned with God. From seven onward, you might experience several Gods sequentially. The God of the seven year old is not the God of the teenager.

At each subsequent stage of life, you redesign your God. In the early twenties, developmental focus is on independence, career, and pair bonding. Breaking away from your family of origin often requires designing a new God that reflects your individuation.

During your thirties, parenting becomes a focus. You may see God differently when you are raising your own children. Then at midlife, another God may meet your needs. Your developmental task is deeper authenticity. A popular question is "Who am I beyond work and family?"

During senior years, your God may become transcendent and less worldly. Your developmental task is to prepare for transition. You may need a new relationship with God to help you bridge the worlds at death.

In addition to developmental changes, your divine and earthly natures have radically different needs. Your earthly nature is physical, emotional, and mental. Your divine nature includes your intuition, Soul, personal God Self, and impersonal God Source.

Your earthly side needs wise parent figures—a Divine Mother and Divine Father. Your Divine Mother is your Soul. She is unconditionally loving and personally involved with your progress. She is an aspect of God. You met her in the Golden Sun training.

Your Divine Father is your personal God Self. You experienced him in the Silver Sun. He is the Light of Truth. He teaches power, detachment, limits, and the law.

Love and Truth—your Soul and your personal God Self—are the parent aspects of God that serve your human evolution. They nurture and develop your earthly nature.

As you evolve spiritually, you discover your divine anatomy. In addition to your Soul and God Self, your divine side requires an impersonal, universal, infinite, and eternal God.

The personal God Self is the highest most humans go on the God Ladder. However, if you are a spiritual initiate or involved in profound healing, you may explore the 7th rung—the impersonal God Source.

The impersonal God goes beyond your mind. Beyond understanding, it cannot be conceived of or spoken about. The impersonal God Source is inscrutable. The prophet Isaiah describes God Source, saying, "My ways are not your ways. My ways are higher than you can see." God's plan for you is unfathomable. Your profound place in the universe is beyond human view. Your God Source is the Great Mystery.

The impersonal God Source—the Void—can be problematic. While your personal God Self is a concept, impersonal God Source is beyond conceptualization. Because it is infinite, eternal, and unchanging, the Void is deconstructed—or you might say, unconstructed. To the rational mind, dematerialization is unfamiliar, suspect, and even hostile territory.

By design, your mind gets you around the earthly world of duality. The mind specializes in subject/object relationships. In the Void, there is neither subject nor object. The mind is in a foreign land. It is inadequate in transcendent, ethereal realms of spirit.

To merge with the Void in ultimate God union, you must transcend your mind. Divine realms require that you go deeper than critical, left-brain thinking. Only faith and spirit suffice at the 7th rung.

Most humans are highly identified with the mind. Leaving the mind behind can be tantamount to self-destruction and death. Accessing the impersonal, universal God Source can be more daunting than climbing Mt. Everest!

Every viewpoint from the God Ladder reveals a new God. Each developmental stage of life creates a new God. None of these divergent views is wrong or incorrect.

When your perspective changes, your experience of God changes. You not only have a new relationship with God, but you also have a new God.

Remember the earlier story where three blind men define an elephant. While each man's description is correct, none has the overall picture. Each man tells his truth from his vantage point. The same multiple-perspectives applies to defining God. Your rendition changes depending upon where your identity focalizes on your God Ladder in any given moment.

It is important to honor and acknowledge all your views of God. None are wrong. Each viewpoint serves a different part of your nature. New understanding arises at each level.

Spiritual growth takes you up the God Ladder. Eventually you anchor your identity in God Source, simultaneously while experiencing your earthly human life.

Who Is Your God?

Know thyself.
—Oracle at Delphi

Clarity regarding your God can speed and strengthen your healing journey. To be happy and healthy, it is important to have a trustworthy God. The following questions help you sort out who your God is and how you relate. You may want to reinvent your God concept and your relationship with God.

Who is Your God?

- When, where, and how do you know God? How do you see, feel, hear, and experience God?
- What activities make you feel close to God? Some people experience God on the greens while golfing. Others feel God in nature while hiking.
- Find an archetype, icon, or symbol that best represents your God. My sister feels closest to God while kayaking. Hers is a River God. My husband's God is the Senior Design Engineer of the Universe.
- Do you humanize God? Or, is your God impersonal?
- How do you define your God? Robin Williams' God is wonder. Abraham Lincoln said, "When I do good, I feel good. When I do

bad, I feel bad. That is my religion." Albert Einstein's God is "the mysterious." Perhaps your God is the universal laws of nature. Some say God is the organizing principle behind all existence. Dr. Deepak Chopra says, "God is the universal, non-local, self-referencing, cybernetic field of energy." Is this your God?

- Do you discern the difference between your personal God and the impersonal, universal, infinite, eternal God Source?
- Which is your favorite: your personal God or the impersonal God Source?
- What does your God do? Is yours a creator God? Destroyer? Preserver?
- What are the limits and powers of your God?
- How does your God feel about time and space? Earthly existence?
- What are the qualities of God? Is your God merciful? Loving? Forgiving? Trustworthy? All-wise? Eternal? Infinite? Unchanging? Powerful? Just? Tyrannical? Punishing? Is your God omnipresent, omniscient, and omnipotent? Is your God male? Female? Neuter? Bi-gendered?
- Which of your parents does your God resemble? Describe the ways in which your God resembles each parent.
- Does God punish you when you are bad and reward you when you are good? What does God do when you are "bad" and "good?"
- Review the developmental periods of your life. Examine your God concept at each stage: childhood, pre-pubescence, teen-ager, young adult, adult, parent, mid-life, senior status.
- Which period of your life most involved you with God? Why?
- Which developmental God do you like best? At what time in life were you happiest with God?
- How is your God different today?
- How does God help you?
- What are your duties to God?
- What are the rules of your relationship?
- What patterns describe your style of connecting with God? Do you connect during crises? Are your God connections self-motivated or does God have to come find you?

- Is there any discomfort in your relationship? Anything you don't like? How would you change your relationship with God? Is there anything missing? What do you want from God that you are not receiving?

- How would you change your God? How must God change to match your pictures?

- Whose God would you prefer? Think of the various Gods in history, cultures, religions, TV, media, and among friends.

- How must you change to be in God alignment?

- Do you argue with God? Do you feel you have the right to tell God what you truthfully think and desire?

- Are you angry with God? Has God let you down? Do you feel betrayed and abandoned by God? Are you alienated from your God? Are you at war with your God?

- Do you try to manipulate God by being "good"? Do you deserve God's love just as you are? Or must you earn God's love?

- Do you feel you "should" receive rewards of health, wealth, and love if you are a good person?

- Does your God love saints more than sinners?

- Do you subtly judge God wrong if you don't receive rewards for your good behavior? Are you setting yourself up as a false-god by judging God?

- Are you walled-off and untrusting of your infinite supply, intelligence, and healing?

- Do you feel cynical or skeptical about God?

- What role does your God play in disease? As a creator? As an observer? Why does God allow pain in your life? Is pain punishment?

- Does God create your destiny or do you have free will?

- How will God function in relation to your death? How will your relationship with God change after you die?

- Do the events of your life align with your concept of God?

- Does God ever disappoint you? How do you deal with God when S/He falls short of your expectations?

- Do you need a referee to help you make peace with God? A therapist? Priest? Minister? Imam? Rabbi? Cleric? Trusted friend?

- Do you trust your God? Is your God trustworthy? Do you totally trust God's plan for you?
- How must you or your God change to restore trust?
- Can you consciously surrender your mind and access your faith?
- Are your values, as you demonstrate them in daily life, congruent with your beliefs about God? Do your thoughts, speech, and actions match your beliefs?
- Which people in your life, history, literature, or media make you feel close to God? Who are the most Godlike people in your life? Who are your models for a healthy, happy God relationship?
- How do you know when your identity is focalized in your physical body? In your emotions? In your mind? In your intuition? In your Soul? In your personal God? In impersonal God Source?
- How does God feel in your body? Your emotions? Your mind? Your intuition? Your Soul? Your spirit? the Void?
- How do you express your love and gratitude to God?
- When, where, and how do you worship God?
- Which of the following describes your primary relationship with God: parent/child, master/servant, tyrant/victim, friend, comforter, counselor, lover, protector, partner, judge, liberator, refuge, regenerator, teacher/mentor/guide?

Reinvent Your God

No more second-hand God.
—Buckminster Fuller

The healing journey creates profound changes in your experience of God. Disease, catastrophe, and pain can create crises of faith. Betrayal and abandonment issues may arise. You may find yourself judging God rather than surrendering.

Revisit the above inventory as you continuously reinvent your God. Remember that God is both immanent and transcendent— personal and impersonal—relative and absolute.

Your earthly self needs an approachable, nurturing personal God that you can talk to at the 6th rung of your God Ladder. Your divine side needs an impersonal, infinite, eternal, unchanging God at the 7th rung. To be whole, it is your job to design both a personal and an impersonal God.

Your 6th rung personal God Self works as a team with your Soul to parent and comfort your earthly self. Your God Self is a manageable form of the universal God. Your personal God Self safely links you to the impersonal infinite Void.

By humanizing and personalizing God, your earthly self can grow—continuously transcending old limits. Eventually, as you transcend your earthly selves, you discover the impersonal, infinite supply of the universal God.

Your deepest healing and regeneration occur when you access the universal God Source. God Source contains infinite supply, intelligence, and healing. Your God Source is ongoing refuge and renewal.

When you know yourself in both earthly and divine realms, you no longer oppositionalize them. By integrating your earthly and divine natures, you bring God to earth. With integration, your identity shifts. You accept life as it is—whether pain or pleasure. You have skills to deal with both heaven and earth.

The hazard of not having access to an absolute God is grandiosity and egotism. Trusting God Source is an irrational act, requiring faith, spiritual IQ, and surrender.

The hazard of not constructing a personal God is that you feel abandoned, alienated, alone, and betrayed. You risk becoming cynical, angry, or depressed.

Reinvent your God in the space below. Design both your personal and your impersonal God.

_____

_____

_____

_____

_____

IDENTITY

All of men's troubles stem from his inability to sit quietly in a room alone.
—Pascal

I am a spiritual being having a human experience.
—Unknown

You are God's self-referencing, cybernetic, feedback loop.
—Deepak Chopra, M. D.

You are God playing in matter.
—Judith Larkin Reno, Ph. D.

Guruji Shows Me Myself

It is the chief point of happiness that a man is willing to be who he is.
—Desiderius Erasmus

On the night Guruji came to visit, I was near death. How did he know when I needed him?

He came into my room, followed by his two brahmacharinis, Sita and Maheshwari. Both young women had taken a lifetime vow of chastity, poverty, and service to Guruji. What a spiritually elegant, noble procession they made.

I felt honored when Guruji took a seat by my bed. We talked about pain and death—how to manage both. While our earth-plane conversation continued, a deeper reality unfolded within me.

Focusing on Guruji, my eyes were unmoving. The room filled with Golden Light. As the meditation deepened, the Light grew so bright, I almost shouted, "Stop! I need sunglasses!"

Instead, I continued my one-pointed gaze, merging deeper into the Light. While simultaneously enjoying a satisfying conversation with Guruji at the earthly level, my spirit soared—bursting into heavenly realms.

On the inner worlds, Guruji showed me a picture of myself. At first, I fought looking. But, he persisted. The picture Guruji projected was not the way I saw myself. Rather, it was the way Guruji saw me— through the eyes of God. He showed me my first picture of my True Self.

She was beautiful. Her essence was love. She was filled with joy.

Disbelieving, I tried to erase the picture and return to earth. However, Guruji's meditative energy was powerful. He held my focus in the Reality of my True Self.

I heard her say, "I am Divine Mother. I am your True Self. I am a regal, mighty force. I am magnanimous, nurturing, unconditionally loving, wise, and untouched by worldly change.

"I am humanity's Silent Witness. I watch the endless pullulation of human life as it weaves and fluctuates. Humans get themselves into fascinating predicaments. However, events that humans deem important, I see as insubstantial. They are interesting entertainment, nothing more.

"I see earthly intrigues as decoration on a cake—a sweet confection, but superficial. Humans take events so seriously. By contrast, I see earthly events as the froth of waves crashing against the beach. Humans are children playing a game with sea foam and frosting!

"As Divine Mother, I adore watching my children. They endlessly delight me. I love them profoundly. Each child is singular and exquisitely beautiful.

"With leonine ferocity, I fix on the divine jewel within each child. I nurture the jewel, holding it in the safety of my heart long enough for it to grow strong.

"I am the one who admires the perfection, everywhere, in everyone, at all times. I am safe harbor in the storm. I reveal the wisdom in the wound. I dry the tears and bring the sun. I am transcendent love. I am Mother of all that is."

As I listened and watched Divine Mother, her beauty surged through me. Her power almost took me away. How strange! I'd rather faint than see the Truth of my Being.

My True Self was shockingly great. I remembered Marianne Williamson's beautiful quote from *A Return to Love,*

> . . . Our deepest fear is not that
> we are inadequate.
> Our deepest fear is that we are
> powerful beyond measure.
>
> It is our Light, not our Darkness,
> that most frightens us.

Throughout my life, I carried a radically smaller self-image than Divine Mother. I hadn't been ready to see my True Self, until now. Despite my Guides repeatedly saying, "Know yourself as God," I hadn't realized their literalness. They had often pointed out, "Your True Self is the Lord God of your being. You are one with your Divine Self."

Prior to Guruji's revelation, I was self-diminishing. I thought I was being spiritual by belittling myself! In actuality, discounting myself was a false defense-mechanism. Self-erasure was a relic from the past when it wasn't safe to be my True Self.

With Guruji, it was safe. He wasn't threatened by my greatness, because he knew his own True Identity—and he understood its right use. With the guru's clarity, he reinforced and affirmed every individual's True Self. Anyone in Guruji's presence was brought to the divine level of being. Anyone who was open and willing could see her own True Self.

Through Divine Mother's eyes, I saw the world engaged in endless posturings—some of them tragic, some hilarious, some victorious, some foolish. I saw events as if through a long-distance lens, with the solid detachment of cosmic perspective. As passionately as I loved, I also had healthy un-caring and holy non-attachment. I could pick events up and put them down. They were extraneous to my identity.

As Divine Mother, I radiated the most glorious love, love, love. It filled my children with life and joy.

Occasionally, one of my children penetrated the thin veil of earthly reality. For a brief instant—awakened from his earthly dream—he peeked through the opening to see me. At that magical moment, I felt like a human mother whose baby first notices her as separate from the background. The first time baby smiles at mother, the mother is overwhelmed with love and pride.

As Divine Mother, I joyously lifted my newly awakened child into the God Light. I showed him the immaculately clear divine realm contrasting with the earthly drama that consumed his mind. I helped him to discern eternal Truth from the passing facts of mundane living. I opened the gateway to his liberation.

As Divine Mother, I enjoyed myself enormously. With an all-knowing Mona Lisa smile, I moved through the many worlds unmoved, solidly anchored in the Great Mystery.

Suddenly, the meditation ended. I jolted back into my sick body. I was back in the narrow, rented hospital bed in my bedroom—back in the philosophical conversation with Guruji at the all-too-human level.

I fluctuated several times, referencing the Golden Light—just to be sure it was real. It was fun flexing my consciousness muscles, moving in and out of higher Reality. I wanted to stay there. However, I knew it was time to return to earth.

Eventually, my interview with Guruji ended. He and his noble entourage filed out of my room. He had come and done his job.

Even though I fought it, he showed me the Truth of my Being. Once you've seen it, you don't forget.

I wondered why it was so difficult for me to see my own Infinite Beauty. Why did I fight the Godness inside my being? I've spent an entire lifetime seeking God, traveling throughout the world. Yet when God revealed herself, why did I run and hide!

To the outside eye, Guruji's visit looked simple and straightforward—a saint doing sickbed duty. How little we know of what we see. Appearance belies the sanctity of everyday events. Guruji's simple, bedside visit left me with my first true glimpse of my Self.

Guruji gave me the gift of myself.

Unmasking

What a thing it is to sit absolutely alone.
—Thomas Merton

Illness has a way of penetrating superficiality and revealing True Self—expeditiously. Unmasking is one of the great services that illness provides.

My beautiful friend Dr. Vivian King is a vitally engaging, skillful, loving teacher. She is also a psychotherapist and an advanced spiritual initiate. She teaches a class called "Masks."

Students make masks representing different aspects of themselves. Masks might symbolize the internal hero, favorite self, anti-hero, rebel, clown, victim, orphan, loser, controller, critic, enemies, or disowned selves. Vivian uses the masks—trading them among students—to unveil the place inside that goes beyond masking.

Behind a mask, I'm at liberty to clown and play the fool. I gain courage and Truth-telling. I can offend or embrace, unleashing whatever mood is in me. The mask liberates fragments of my Soul, moving them into action so I can see them.

Confidence builds that says, "What will happen if I drop the mask? What lies behind the mask? Who am I without the mask?"

The class deepens to a quiet place. We experience the common bond of our humanity. With the shallows explored, we are ready to plumb deeper waters.

A master teacher like Vivian unveils the place behind the masks. In the deep unmasking, there is no pretense, no push, or pull. We absorb into the silence, without a need to speak.

In the silence, Vivian reveals the place that never moves at the bottom of the sea—regardless of surface waves and disturbances. She energetically connects us to the unchanging power of our Infinite Core.

Illness performs a similar service of unmasking. In fact, it is the master class of unmasking! Disease demands that I go deeper than my chemo-styled baldness and steroid swollen face.

I must penetrate many masks. My skin sprouts plastic lumens and polyurethane tubing. Where is my old, familiar body? I learn that I am not my body.

My beloved, ancient body parts no longer move. I discover that I am not freedom or movement.

Increased weight morphs me into unwieldy foreign shapes. I am so fragile that it is dangerous to turn over in bed. I gradually understand that I am not my form or powers.

Who am I underneath all the masks of the external world? Without the elegant body parts and great makeup, who am I? Who am I beyond disease labels, medical paraphernalia, and endless treatments? What part of me survives beyond the endgame?

Illness performs a mighty service. It liberates me from superficial show and external performance. There's nothing to do now. Nowhere to go. The masks come off.

It is the soothing undoing, when dusk undoes the shape and form of things, disrobing the day. No longer distracted, I go deeper into the night to touch a more authentic self than could be revealed by sight.

Illness tolerates no mask. I go beyond vulnerability to the unmoved Strength of God that I am. I go beyond worldly facts to my unchanging inner Truth. Illness has brought me to the door of eternity. Who will I be on the other side? What mighty force has delivered me here?

What is this penetrating honesty that illness brings? There is no longer room for pretty posturing or primping. Illness drills a hole to more solid ground. It necessitates Truth.

Without strength to hold them up, I must drop the masks.

Don't Confuse Your Identity with Pain

If you understand, things are just as they are. If you do not understand,
things are just as they are.
—Zen Proverb

Don't let pain devour your identity. With all the medical intensity, life-and-death decisions, crises, problem solving, and emergency hospital admissions, your own drama may trap you. Step back to gain perspective.

You are not the first to deal with pain and medical procedures, even imminent death. Pain comes to everyone. Death comes with the birth certificate. Don't take your life personally!

Pain can collapse your self-worth, as it robs your worldly roles. There may be days when you can't pay the bills or return important phone calls. Even bathing can become an impossible task. The pain can be so great, that important worldly responsibilities become nothing.

Rather than rob you, let pain teach you how to disidentify with worldly things. Let it unmask you, giving you distance from your life. Let it liberate you from your old identities. Go deeper. Discover who you are without all the worldly trappings.

Instead of fixating on pain and loss, focus on your God Source. Become absorbed in the Silence, even while pain hammers you. Remember the part of you that is Untouched. Go beneath the agonizing fluctuations of pain waves to the Immovable Place at the bottom of the ocean.

Your problems are ocean waves, disturbances on the surface. Waves are guaranteed to break. Don't confuse daily disturbances with the clear Deep Source of your being.

During crisis, repeat this chant:

I am not my body.
I am not my emotions.
I am not my thoughts.
I am that which is greater.

I am not the negative.
I am not the pain.
I am Infinite Supply, God Divine.

Remember Walt Whitman saying, "I am large. I contain multitudes."

Long bouts with pain and disease teach who you are and who you are not. Pain is contractive. If you identify with pain, you shrink into oblivion. Don't confuse your identity with your pain.

Instead, use pain as a landmark showing who you are not. Go in the opposite direction to find your expansive, limitless True Self. Say to yourself, "I am not pain. I am that which is greater."

Find the part of you that is untouched by pain. There is an absolute level of Reality where you are unmoved. This is your True Self.

To find your True Self, discover where your earthly self begins and ends. When you follow your human self back to its source, there is a point where human reality dissolves. It becomes meaningless. This is the point of transcension and God union.

Through transcension, you are free. It is a great ally when you are working with pain. Transcension brings you home to your True Self. It liberates you from the time/space box, while you are simultaneously living in the box.

Rely on your True Self. Cultivate a relationship with it. Sometimes, the pain is so great that just knowing another realm exists saves you!

Knowing who you are and who you are not is essential in the journey through pain and disease. You are not your pain or disease. While recuperating from colon cancer, Ronald Reagan said, "I didn't' have cancer, something inside me had cancer and it was removed." He had identified who he was and who he was not.

Your True Self is found in the stillness beyond pain. Your True Self is the space between the stars, the gap between thoughts, the stop between the inhale and the exhale, the silence between the notes, the screen behind the movie.

To discover your True Self, try figure-ground reversal. Look into the emptiness, rather than the form. Practice seeing the space around objects as defining them. For example, the cup is empty space in a particular shape. Practice valuing the emptiness.

To discover your True Self, lie on the ground. As clouds move across the sky, focus your eyes in a diffused, broadened gaze until you can see the entire sky behind the changing clouds.

Know the sky as the screen of your being, your True Self. Practice discerning between the sky and clouds in your life. Move your focus from transitory earthly events to your divine True Self.

Pain forces you to keep the company of the holy. To preserve your sanity, pain demands that you develop refuge in God.

Buddha saw suffering in the world. He realized it is possible to be non-attached to pain. He didn't confuse his identity with his pain.

Ultimately, pain delivers you to your True Identity. Through the process of elimination, you discover who you are and who you are not. Or, is that the process of illumination!

I Am the Space Between the Stars

O Thou Self revealing One,
Reveal Thyself in me.
—Sanskrit Prayer

Here are some identity shifts and gifts that I received from my healing journey. Searching for my True Identity amidst the pain, I continuously ask, "Who am I?" To find my essence, I must discover what remains after removing all the roles and masks in my life. What is unchanging and irreducible within me?

- I am the Silence, the unmoving screen behind the activities of my life. Sri Poonja says, "You came from the Silence. You will return to the Silence. It is your fundamental self."
- I am infinite and eternal. No earthly events can damage my True Self.

- I am universal. My healing journey is part of God's universal plan. My personal journey serves the universe in ways that I may never understand.
- I am absolute and immovable. Despite mundane appearances, my True Self is unchanged.
- I am perfect, regardless of external appearances.
- I am one with everything. Other people's beauty, joys, and victories are mine.
- I am God in human form. Through me, God sees, enjoys, and becomes his creation. I am God infusing spirit into matter. I am God evolving matter into spirit. The more conscious, empty, and clear I become, the easier it is for God to see, act, and be through me. I provide quite a service for God!
- The fabric of earthly consciousness is the thinnest of veils, which I penetrate with my mind. Once free, I am absorbed into the luminescent ground of being through mindlessness. I use my mind to transcend my mind.
- Behind the rock, cloud, and horse, I see the golden glow of God's face. God's luminescence pulses and throbs through all manifest form.
- I am the living love, the Light Divine.
- Continuing further in my journey Home, behind God's luminescence is the Fertile Void. It is everywhere, in everything—in objects and in space.
- I am infinite Potential and dynamic Peace.
- I am infinite healing, energy, intelligence, and supply.
- Divine Light and God Sound are stepping-stones guiding me Home to my origin, the Fertile Void.
- "I am a water bird flying into the sun."—Jelaluddin Rumi
- I am the space between the stars.

GRIEF

Your grief is a hand mirror held up to where you are doing
your best work.
—Jelaluddin Rumi

Sow in tears; reap in joy.
—Hebrew Saying

Grieve it and get over it. Move on!
—Judith Larkin Reno, Ph. D.

When to Fold 'Em

The function of healthy grief is to make space for new life and
new identity.
—Judith Larkin Reno, Ph. D.

Grief is a birthing process. Through the labor pains of grief, you give birth to your new identity. You get another chance to confront the darkness, forgive ignorance, transcend, and rescript your life at a new and higher level.

Grief insists that you walk away from the past. You must trust that the future will be better, despite apparent loss. Faith teaches you to look deeper, beneath the surface of events. Faith is in the unseen. Trusting God's perfect plan affirms that the future will be better, no matter what your mind says.

Through healthy grieving, you reframe each loss to a triumph. You discover the gift of growth that adversity provides. Valuing God's will beyond your own, you surrender your negative judgments. You focus on God's gift rather than on your loss.

In healthy grieving, you hold your sacrifice inside your heart as one of life's treasures. Without transmutation skills, you could falsely believe your loss was God's condemnation. You could think of yourself as a victim, forgetting that you created your Soul Contract. You could forget that whatever happens could not be otherwise.

In Reality, there is no loss. All of life's victories are yours forever. No one can ever take away your experience of love, for example. This belongs to you and no one else. It is your treasure—a gift from God. Emphasize the gift rather than the loss.

The sooner you emphasize the gift rather than the loss, the better you will feel. Treasure hunt for the wisdom gift in painful emotions, false beliefs, and physical pain. Don't allow grief to accumulate. Keep transmuting it into treasure.

Always insist on a better future, even if that means making peace with death. When you're facing death, instead of dwelling on what you're losing, focus on harvesting the triumphs of a lifetime. Learn about the gifts, freedoms, and powers beyond death. Embrace a glorious future, even as you say goodbye to the past.

As toddlers, we learn two basic life skills: to open and close, to contract and release. The toddler learns to open and close his hand. He picks things up and puts them down. Potty training teaches him to hold and release.

Life goes in endless cycles of opening and closing, expanding and contracting, holding and releasing. Grief teaches the emotional muscle of release.

In life, you know that all things have an end. You increase your power when you release the past with dignity. As Kenny Rogers sings, "Know when to hold 'em and know when to fold 'em."

When you get sick, it seems as if you are losing everything. You see your life and everything you value slip away. Your plans for the future evaporate. Your sense of self disappears. Your standing in the world is marginalized. Your goals become meaningless. Who you were in the past is gone. Your new identity is not clear yet.

Grieving demands that you move through denial, anger, depression, and sorrow to arrive at acceptance of your loss. Acceptance is easier if you can trust God and find the gift of wisdom in your loss.

Always go toward the gain rather than away from the pain. What are you learning through the pain? What are the new gifts of spirit in your healing journey? What are your new powers? What is your new awareness?

Reframe your loss, emphasizing the positive. After all, you are lucky you had something to lose! Many people never experience the joys of love, success, prosperity, family, ownership, health, happiness, intelligence, spirit, or freedom. It is a skill to translate whatever is lost into a sacred memory, a triumph for your Treasure Box.

When grief shows up, use your will to choose the positive. Look at the gift and the victory instead of the loss. Remember Helen Keller saying, "When the door of happiness closes, another opens; but often we look so long at the closed door that we do not see the one which has opened for us."

Grief as Shape-Shifter

> *Often when you're at the end of something, you're at the*
> *beginning of something else.*
> —Mr. Fred Rogers

The great thirteenth century Sufi poet Jelaluddin Rumi comments on grief as a shamanic shape-shifter. Grief liberates you from one form to another, one earthly identity to another. Grief cracks you open, again and again. Gradually, you understand you are none of the forms.

Eventually, grief helps you attend to God, the great presence behind all forms. Through grief, you transcend form and merge with God. An old American proverb says, "Freedom is when you have nothing left to lose." Grief is a path to spiritual liberation!

Rumi says, "Don't grieve. Anything you lose comes around in another form." I would add, be careful you don't confuse any of the forms with your Ultimate Identity. The nature of earthly life is illusory shape-shifting.

The ultimate gift of grief is transcension and liberation from form into God union.

WILL TO LIVE

I think I can. I think I can. I think I can.
—Watty Piper, *The Little Engine That Could*

Reinvent Your Will to Live

We begin again, all compassionate, loving Oneness. Bismilla.
—Islam

In surviving serious illness, your sheer will to live is a powerful ally. As the Russian proverb says, "Pray to God, but row for shore."

At each new level of healing, you may need to reinvent your reason for living. Every time you cycle-up in your healing, you walk into a foreign country. You learn a new language of ideas, values, and sense of self. There are often new problems to solve involving diet, exercise, doctors, and medicines. It can be tempting to give up the struggle, especially when you are in one of these threshold experiences.

Fighting to live can be disorienting. Sometimes you don't know if you're coming or going! Doing what it takes to stay here requires repeated firm resolve.

To strengthen your resolve, periodically self-interview to find your reasons for living. What do you live for? Why is it worth fighting to live? Who or what keeps you here? What is still undone in your life? What do you want to experience or complete before you leave? What motivates your fight to live?

Be specific in your interview. Keep searching until you think, "That's it! That's why the struggle is worth it. I'm living for_____." You fill in the blank.

You might have several reasons to stay alive. List them in order of priority. Your reasons for living can change from one healing cycle to the next.

Don't take your will to live for granted. During catastrophic illness, you must continuously regenerate your will to live. It is like a muscle. Exercise it every day.

To increase your clarity, write your reasons for living. Writing demands clarity. Clarity is the first step in manifestation.

I learned about the power of clarity through my dear friend, Lisa. She went on a power journey, deep inside the Ecuadorian Amazon jungle, where she worked with four shamans. She took a scroll with prayers to give each healer. My name was on her healing scroll. I said, "I pray for complete healing so I may dance with joy, peace, and love on earth."

When Lisa asked me to summarize my prayer into one line, it focused my clarity. Clarity cuts through the fog and connects you with your perfect future. What prayer would you put on the healing scroll?

To further clarify your reasons for living, examine different areas of your life. For example, my will to live generates from my love for my husband, family, friends, and work. I treasure playing the violin, teaching, counseling, writing, reading, learning, and nature hikes. These are the great gifts of my life. They motivate me in the daily battle to live. I reference them frequently throughout the day.

Doing medical procedures forty hours plus per week is difficult work! I need a prize to reward my hard work. Knowing exactly why I am willing to endure pain to attain health focuses me. I keep my eye on the prize, rather than on the pain.

In assessing your will to live, quality of life is important. Endless suffering in terminal disease is of little value. There must be pleasure in life. Periodically, assess your pleasure/pain balance. Each person's pleasure/pain balance is different. How much pain are you willing to endure in order to live? What are your limits? How much pain will you endure before you will be willing to die?

When I was so near death, I went to the other side and looked back at life. I kept switching views: living/dying; human side/ graduation; staying/going. There were values on both sides.

On the other side, there was no physical pain. I was free of the time/space box. I could reunite with old friends who graduated before me. I could teach and study the mystical subjects I love.

However, for me the Light was on the human side. Suddenly, I realized, "Most of the people I love are here!" I can more easily help them if I have a physical body. I can teach and study mysticism here as well.

Each person has a different experience finding the will to live. When you open door #1 marked EARTH LIFE, look inside and see what your future life on earth can offer. Then, open door #2 marked LIFE ON THE OTHER SIDE. Ask your Guides to show you images and feelings of your life after death.

On which side do you feel more fulfilled, liberated, and complete? On which side do you feel more love? More joy? More learning? Where is your desire—on the side of earth life or on the other side?

What are your reasons for living? Why do you fight to live? **List your reasons for living below:**

_____
_____
_____
_____
_____

Find the Healing Path

About the only difference between stumbling blocks and
stepping stones is the way you use them.
—Bernard Meltzer, M. D.

When I was in the darkest hours, my daughter Sara said, "There is a way out, Mom. There's always a way out. The Healing Path is there. Other people have walked it. Other people have received terminal diagnoses and lived. Anastasia's sister lived thirty years after they told her she only had days and weeks left.

"There is a way to complete healing. You can find it too, Mom. Find the Healing Path. It's there. Feel it, Mom. Do you see it? Do you see the Path out of pain? It leads back to life."

I did see it. First, I saw it from an aerial view. The Path lit up. It glowed like a trickle of hot, gold lava winding through dark mountain ranges. The gold slit of hot Light looked up at me with an otherworldly wisdom.

I traced its serpentine progress over jagged-toothed rocks and through precipitous mountain climbs. The trail disappeared behind ominous, jutting peaks. There were abrupt switchbacks. The Healing Path was thin-lipped, with thousand foot drops just inches from each foothold.

"Yeowza!" I thought. "I'm supposed to hike this! As much as I love hiking, maybe I'll pass."

Despite treacherous footing, the trail did cross the summit. It came out the other side of the dark wilderness.

I could see the end of it! The trail gently descended to the other side of the mountain. The lush green valley below radiated joy, love, peace, healing, and vitality. The Great Light of Life pulsed in the valley at the end of the grueling hike.

Sara insisted, "Do you see it, Mom? Do you see the Path back to life?"

I had to admit, I did see it. I avoided mentioning to Sara how closely the word "trail" resembles "trial."

Sara continued enthusiastically, "Now, go to the beginning of the trail. Notice how it splits into two pathways, close to the trailhead. One path is dark and dusky. Notice how many people line up for that trail. Find the other path that is bright with Light."

Back on the ground, my job was more difficult than from the aerial view. Threading among the crowd, eventually I found the beginning of the Lighted Path. There were fewer people there. The energy was difficult and intense.

By contrast, the dark path was flat and unchallenging. It was the more popular of the two choices. Clearly, it would have been an easier option for someone in my condition. However, I slogged ahead to the Lighted trailhead.

I took my place on the Healing Path. Immediately, the otherworldly Light locked onto me with blinding intensity. Its tangible force practically flattened me.

Slowly, I adjusted to its enormous power. The Light was a laser from some unseen horizon—far ahead. It defined the trail.

The Light had unspeakable, unremitting presence. It drove me and everyone on the Path toward our goal of healing. Healing was truly the Light at the end of our tunnel.

It required tunnel vision to persevere in the grueling, healing march. A powerful will to live motivated each of us. With blinders and singleness of purpose, we trudged past many fallen bodies beside the trail.

Silhouettes ahead of me outlined the dignity of each marcher's bearing. They held their heads high with their eyes riveted on the Light. Rhythmically and robotically, we walked as if in a deep trance. We were determined to remain merged with the Light in our return to life. The intensity of each hard-won step revealed the serious, survival nature of our procession.

After walking for a while, I noticed everyone in line ahead of me was bald, just like me. The voice of my Inner Guide said, "All these people are bald from their cancer treatments. Like you, they are fighting to live. They will succeed. They have found the Lighted Path. Follow them. Copy them. Think of nothing else.

"Whatever disaster your medical tests indicate or the doctors predict, pretend they are speaking in a foreign language that does not concern or affect you. You stay concentrated on the Light on the Path.

"Keep walking in the line, one step at a time. Think only of your next step. You **will** have your life back. You have found the Healing Path."

Stairway to Heaven

> *It is our attitude at the beginning of a difficult undertaking*
> *which more than anything else, will determine its outcome.*
> —William James

When you hang out at Death's Door, everyone in your love circle gets a wake-up call. It is said that you don't know what a person means to you until they die.

One of the blessings of the cancer journey is that I had time to say good-bye to everyone. I watched the changes in my loved ones as they fought for my life and dealt with the possibility of losing me.

My daughter Sara lives in Hawaii. She is almost six feet tall, beautiful, and fun-loving. She's large-boned, muscular, strong, and athletic. I told her, "You're like a nuclear reactor. You're extra powerful. You need to be careful how you use your power so you don't scare people. Other people don't have your power. Be gentle with that great power of yours." During my healing journey, she used her power to heal me.

When I was near death, Sara came to the mainland to visit for ten days. In the past, she had been irresponsible with her time commitments. Usually, if she set an appointment, I allowed an hour for her to be late. Sometimes, she didn't show up at all.

On this visit, she matured. I watched her turn into a woman. She was deeply motivated to help me and to be with me. She showed up at my side every day and wasn't late for a single appointment.

Many days, I was too weak to speak. However, Sara was undaunted. She sat silently with me for hours, radiating her healing love. Other people got embarrassed when I was too weak to entertain them. However, Sara was not there for the social event. She just wanted to love me.

If I fell asleep, Sara continued shining her healing love on me. All her life, I called her my "Sunshine." When Sara was born, the sun came out in my life. Sitting beside me during my illness, she felt like a healing sun.

Because she is so physical, during her visit I wanted Sara to have a place to put her energy. She knows I love to hike in the woods. Since my illness, I had been too weak to stand up much, let alone hike. But, in our tiny backyard, we do have our one Tree.

Sara built me a "Stairway to Heaven." It wraps around Tree. On strong days, I can climb the earth stairs and visit my friend,

Tree. I may not be able to walk in the woods, but I can walk in the wood!

Sara put a chair at the top of the stairway behind Tree, so I can go there and meditate. I can pretend I'm in the forest. Positive fantasy is an important survival skill!

Every day, Sara brought a different gift to surprise me. She brought beautiful polished shells from Hawaii, so I could hear the ocean. One perfect, hot-pink, conch shell spiraled with delicate, fragile points. She carried it three thousand miles without losing a single tip. I touched each perfect pink tip.

Sara brought food and cooked for us. Her flowers decorated the table.

We sat in the waning sunlight of late afternoon watching the birds take golden dust-baths on the new Stairway to Heaven. Curious about the new construction in their neighborhood, the birds fully acquainted themselves with every detail. Clearly pleased, they gabbed simultaneously about their discoveries.

As we watched the bird show, Sara's helium balloons in various shapes floated around the room. They peopled the place with delightful, new energy.

Sara brought new life. Despite excruciating pain, I didn't waste her gifts. I harvested every happy moment and renewed my will to live.

Sunshine Jump-Starts My Life

Lead me, Oh Lord, from death to life.
—Sanskrit

One night toward the end of Sara's visit, I had a lucid dream. Sara led me through a noble, high-canopied forest of redwoods. Dramatic spotlights of holy radiance rayed through the forest, creating a cathedral of Light.

We arrived at a clearing deep inside the forest. The oval meadow dazzled with White Light. The Light polished the surrounding leaves into a reflective, metallic shine.

In the center of the clearing, I saw a Crystal Table constructed of simple lines. The Table was alive, almost like a person, breathing with pulsating Light. Its life came from other worlds. I knew I was to lie on this unusual Table to receive healing.

Three beautiful Beings appeared at my head. Each wore a white robe with a long gold rope tied at the waist. Iridescent Light shined from the fabric of their robes as they moved around me.

These were clearly intergalactic healers of high stature—two women and a man. My Guide said Sara had traveled across the universe to find these particular specialists. They were famous for helping people in my condition.

These expert healers created an electric arc with their hands. It jump-started my brain, restoring my will to live. I was so depleted, they repeated the procedure three times until they reached the appropriate level, pulling me back from death to life.

Ancient Tibetan teaching says all physical healing begins with the heart. To regenerate my heart, the intergalactics placed healing compresses at strategic energy points throughout my body.

Magical flowers and healing herbs unknown on earth composed the healing poultices. They revitalized my knees, legs, hips, forehead, and various other energy points. All the points were essential to healing my heart.

Sara and my other daughter Caitlin stood at my knees. They worked with special compresses to bring vital force into my legs and feet. Revitalizing the legs also restores the will to live. Sara and Cait anchored me on earth, invigorating my will to step forward into new life.

The healing team worked all night. When I woke, I was a different person. I was freshly made and shining with new vitality.

Sara came to visit that day. I told her of the healing dream. She said, "Mom, I had the same dream!"

One of my dear friends, Tera is a powerful healer. She called me the same day. She said, "Judith, every time I come to heal you in the dream worlds, Sara is there. She stations her energy like a bodyguard, protecting you. Nobody can get through to see you without Sara's permission. She is a powerful protector for you!"

In talking with Tera, I realized what a profound healing I had received. I also realized the power of lucid dreaming to heal. Lucid dreaming opens valuable portals of infinite supply, intelligence, and renewal from other worlds. Tera, my children, and I, all had used lucid dreaming for my healing benefit.

Sara had brought the sunshine at other times in my life. Once again, she brought new life.

Waking Up

> *Waking up this morning, I smile.*
> *Twenty-four brand new hours are before me.*
> —Chan Phap Dang, *A Joyful Path*

> *This is the day that the Lord has made; let us rejoice and be*
> *glad in it.*
> —*Psalms 118: 24*

When you face major illness, it takes willpower just to wake up in the morning. The song says, "Breaking up is hard to do." In my case, waking up was hard to do. The moment I regained earthly consciousness, I flooded with the hopelessness of my situation. Waking up each day was a nightmare.

I remembered Rumi saying, "We wake empty and afraid." I was terrified of yet another medical procedure. I said to my husband, "You go in my place. I can't do it."

Gradually, I flagged the problem of waking up and developed strategies to combat my daily dread. I learned to renew my will to live each day. Here are some of the skills I developed.

Before I get out of bed, I turn dread into gratitude—even if I must force myself to be grateful. Upon awakening, I ask my heart to "look for news of love," as Hafiz recommends.

I consciously focus on each blessing in my life: my beloved husband, my family, and my friends. I'm grateful that I can see, hear, smell, taste, touch, and feel emotions. I'm thankful for my mind, spirit, and every working body part. I treasure each functioning part. I don't take them for granted.

Greeting the day with gratitude is a rigor. The great Lebanese poet Kahlil Gibran said, "Wake at dawn and give thanks for another day of loving." If all my other powers are gone, I still have my power to love!

With an act of will, I stay centered in gratitude. I remember how painful it is to fall out of love with life. There is a price to pay if I forget gratitude as my ally. My Inner Guides frequently repeat, "You lose your way if you lose your gratitude."

Healing begins with gratitude. I use gratitude rigors to strengthen my spirit to face the day. Spirit fights pain.

To further strengthen my spirit, I invoke my Soul Council, saying "Surround, guide, and protect me throughout this day." I think of all the allies who will help me during the day: my medical team, friends, family, angels, Spirit Guides, TV friends, books, movies, audio tapes.

I consciously commit to positive thinking throughout the day. I rehearse my positive attitude before getting out of bed. I visualize myself meeting each situation with God as my partner. Imagining how Jesus and the saints would handle each challenge, I model myself after their leadership.

I begin renewing my spirit the previous night. Upon falling asleep, I bless the coming day. I see it held in Golden Light. I visualize Angels of Love, Joy, Healing, and Compassion walking with me through every second of the new day. They roll out a Golden Carpet of love and peace before every step I take.

I visualize myself walking on the Golden Carpet through the entire new day. Wherever I am, God is. With the help of the angels, I set the day up for success.

After strengthening my spirit and before getting out of bed, I inventory the pain. Morning pain can be the worst, before pain meds start. I identify both old and new pains.

I play a game. Whichever body part has the most pain wins the prize. I actually give it a prize in my mind. Like the game-show host, I mentally say, "Come on down! Receive your prize!" This strange ritual helps me retrieve my power from the pain.

Then, I inventory body parts that work and those that don't. Each day is different. With bone cancer, bones migrate in the night. I can have a completely new construction in the morning. Before I navigate getting out of bed, I see what's left of me. Moving slowly in the bed, I make my assessment.

Comedian George Carlin describes growing old. He heroically pries his eyelids open in the morning. Exploring what parts of his face still work, he adds popping sounds to each victory. With ferocious will and bulging eyeballs, he accomplishes the gargantuan task of keeping his eyes open!

Following his lead, I fantasize my getting out of bed as a comedy routine. I hear ridiculous commentary and sound effects in my mind. Laughing at my foolish antics to regain standing in the new day, I say, "She's up. She's down. She's up. Or is she? Yes, there she goes!! Reno's rising. A small step for mankind, a huge step for this woman!"

Sitting on the edge of the bed, I remember the date. Though this sounds mundane, it is very important. When you are lost in a maze of pain and medical procedures, it's easy to lose track of time. I don't allow apparent tragedy to rob me.

To take back my life, I say, "This is the day which the Lord has made for me. There is no other day like it. It is a gift from God. This is my (month) and (day)." I repeat the numbers of the date, consciously visualizing them. I shape the numbers in the air, several times before getting out of bed.

This date ritual ensures that I am present in my day—fully appreciating that this day is mine. It is fresh and precious—beyond any pain it might contain. My identity extends beyond my challenges. I am greater than my body. No illusion of lack will rob me from appreciating the gift of life I have today.

I remember the day of the week and consciously engage with its essence. What does Sunday mean to me? Monday? Tuesday? Wednesday? Thursday? Friday? Saturday? I consciously invest each day of the week with special meaning. I will not sacrifice my days of the week just because they contain medical procedures. Each day brings me closer to healing.

I imagine today's date, along with the day of the week, written on a twelve-inch red Valentine Box—like a box of Valentine candy, with white lace and red satin curled around the edges of the heart. I hold the Valentine close to my heart saying, "This is my day, just for me. This is a gift. I appreciate it!"

I dispassionately survey the medical and physical challenges awaiting me. I see an armada of sacred support walking beside me throughout the day. Together, there is nothing we can't handle.

My real focus today is on finding the treasures in the day. I think of the triumphs I will feel by day's end. I imagine my Harvest Necklace full and glowing. I laugh as if God and I have a special secret. It only looks as if this day is about medical procedures. My real day is about my secret Necklace!

A beautiful, five-thousand-year-old Sanskrit poem "Salutation to the Dawn" inspires me.

Look to this day,
For it is life, the very life of life.
In its brief course
Lie all the verities of your existence;
The bliss of growth;
The glory of action;
The splendor of beauty.
For yesterday is but a dream,
And tomorrow is only a vision.
But today, well lived,
Makes every yesterday a dream of happiness,
And every tomorrow a vision of hope.
Look well, therefore, to this day.
For it is the Beginning of the Dawn.

After getting out of bed, I face the sun and say, "Thank you for my life, Great Spirit. Thank you for my life, Great Spirit. Thank you for my life, Great Spirit."

I don't take a new day of life for granted. With poet John Seed, I pray, "O stars, lend me your burning passion"—so that I may live another day.

The Four-Armed Human Hug

> *With the help of my God, I shall leap over the wall.*
> *—Book of Common Prayer*

Unexpected events can renew your will to live. Shortly after my diagnosis, my daughter Caitlin became pregnant. My sitting in the jaws of death—trying to keep from being devoured each day—contrasted sharply with the new life coming to our family. British poet Tennyson said, babies come "trailing clouds of glory" straight from God. I felt a jolt of new life with this baby.

When Cait and I visit, there is a lot of love between us. Hugging good-bye, I often feel love pouring from our hearts. One night as we hugged good-bye, I felt the usual river of love coming to me. To my surprise, there was a second river of love coming from Cait's abdomen.

When I looked psychically, I saw two tiny arms reaching out to hug me. My yet unborn grandson had enjoyed the love pouring from his mom. He wanted to be part of it. So, he copied his mother's love stream.

Then, he noticed me. His love became personal and even more powerful. I was amazed at the strength of his focus.

I wondered, who is this astonishing Soul coming to me? What powerful past lives have we shared to be so familiar to each other? How is his birth restoring me to life?

This was the first four-armed human hug I ever received. Until then, I didn't know it was possible.

Now, I have received two.

DEATH AS AN IDENTITY CRISIS

We're both alive. For all I know that's what hope is.
—Henry II, *Lion in Winter*

The goal of all life is death.
—Sigmund Freud, Psychotherapist

I shall die. But that is all I will do for death.
—Edna St. Vincent Millay

When death comes, I don't end. The world ends.
—Ayn Rand

Break the surly bonds of earth To touch the face of God.
—John Guillespie McGee, Jr., "High Flight"

There are lands of the living and the dead.
The bridge between them is love.
—Judith Larkin Reno, Ph. D.

When you die, you pass into other people's hearts.
—Billy Joel, Musician and Song Writer

In answer to a student's question: What is death?
Where does the song go when it is sung?
Where does the movie go after it is seen?
—Judith Larkin Reno, Ph. D.

Today could be the last day of the rest of your life.
—Judith Larkin Reno, Ph. D.

Nothing concentrates the mind like the hangman's noose.
—Benjamin Franklin

Death is a horizon. The horizon is nothing, but the limit of our sight . . .
What the Lord gives, nothing can take away . . . The spirit returns to
God who gave it.
—Wesley Carr, Dean of Westminster Cathedral

At death, I will unite with my Light Body Triumphant.
—Judith Larkin Reno, Ph. D.

I'm going to join the Immensity.
—Omar Sharif's character on his death bed, *Monsieur*
Ibrahim

Fear of Death

I'm not afraid of dying. I just don't want to be there when it
happens.
—Woody Allen

Does the wave racing toward the beach look to its left and right
and shriek, "Look out! We're going to crash! We're all going to die!"
Or, is it curious and exhilarated as it surges toward extinction? The
wave seems to know there is no death. It enjoys the process of
changing form and merging once again with the great power of the
ocean.

Does the cloud howl and shrink back, resisting its natural gestation
and extinction when it becomes rain? Or does it enjoy the ride from
sailing the sky, to bursting open, to falling, to merging with the earth,
to evaporating, to forming a cloud, to starting the process all over
again? Is the cloud proud of its shape-shifting talent? Does it relish its
ability to change forms?

What about the sunflower, giving its all to open full-strength and blossom? Does it nit-pick and complain along the way? Is it beleaguered with worries that some day it will disintegrate and become mulch? Who is to say which form is better, the flower or the rich earth it becomes?

Where is my childlike sense of discovery when it comes to death? Where is the enchantment? Why can't I just relax and enjoy the ride? Why must I be so judgmental about changing form on the final ride back to spirit?

I like the story of the monk being chased by a tiger. The monk runs over hill and gully, dodging and outsmarting the tiger. Narrowly escaping the tiger's huge white teeth at every turn, the monk runs to save his life.

The monk runs, even through his exhaustion—until the tiger corners him on a narrow precipice. Balanced on the brink of extinction, the monk feels the tiger's hot breath.

The monk begins falling into the canyon. Suddenly, he catches hold of a root emerging from the side of the cliff. Clinging to the root, he looks up into the gaping jaws of the drooling tiger.

The root holds him momentarily, but the monk knows he is destined to fall. At the last second, he notices a strawberry plant growing from the side of the cliff. The bright red fruit is ripe and luscious. The monk savors its sweet fragrance. Reaching out, he grabs the delicious berry.

He eats it—thoroughly enjoying it—as he falls.

This monk lived until he died. He knew how to be here, now. He truly lived—through all life's changes—without judgmentalness. His sense of enchantment never died.

How Do You Know the Unknowable?

You have to know that death is for the body and that you are
That which will never die.
—Sri Poonja, *The Truth Is*

Spiritual intelligence transcends and exceeds all other forms of intelligence.
—Judith Larkin Reno, Ph. D.

How do you know the Unknowable? The answer is through meditation, prayer, and faith. You know God, not through your mind, but through your spirit.

Cultivating your spiritual intelligence constructs a bridge to life beyond death. The destination of the death experience is God union. Through spiritual intelligence, you ascend your God Ladder and travel to the Mind of God. You are hard-wired to do the journey.

You can't escape your spirit. Your adamantine, diamond spirit is indestructible. Through spirit, you navigate the bardos at death. Through spirit, you unite with the Clear White Light.

As Saint Paul said, "Your faith shall make you whole." There is a science of faith. Death helps you find it.

My Experience Beyond the Bardos

Our death is a wedding with eternity.
—Rumi

As a spiritual teacher, I had studied the process of dying. Different traditions describe the death experience according to their various mythologies.

The Christian tradition describes meeting St. Peter at the Pearly Gates, guarding the entrance to Heaven. The Buddhists work with the Clear White Light as a guide to the higher worlds after death. Dr. Raymond Moody, in his clinical research of near-death experiences, describes progressing through a tunnel when life closes.

Tibetan Buddhists call dying, bardo work. They have an elaborate system of the different worlds, or bardos, you pass through after death. Much of Tibetan bardo work involves moving through your psycho-mental debris as it detoxifies from your incarnation at death. Death is a purification from your life attachments.

To jockey through the debris field of unresolved addictions, desires, angers, sorrows, and fears requires focus. Negative worlds can seduce you with their demons and attractions.

The Tibetan Book of the Dead says, "Be neither attracted nor repulsed," as you travel through the bardos. You must remain detached. Concentrate on the Clear White Light beyond the bardos.

If you can't focus on the Clear White Light, try to remember God. Call angels to help you. Even if you don't feel their presence, they will come. Trust. All will be well. The long, choppy bardo-ride does have an end.

Bardo work is the great unraveling of the lifetime releasing its baggage. In the end, all that remains is your impenetrable, adamantine, pure, diamond spirit. Beyond the bardos is God union, rapturous love, dynamic peace, and freedom.

Some traditions say all spiritual practice is preparation for death. Good bardo work is passing your final exam. It determines your placement after life and your standing in your next life. Some say your death determines whether you transcend the wheel of reincarnation. Unresolved desires and repulsions can bind you to another incarnation.

In his beautiful film *Fierce Grace,* Ram Dass describes his bout with death during his stroke. He experiences self-judgment when he doesn't have a flashy death encounter. He forgets to chant, or visualize White Light, or breathe, or consecrate, or aspire, or even remember God. There are no flashing lights or angels.

Instead, he is present in his body. He observes the ceiling tile rather than celestial denizens. Where are the bardos, the Lights, the tunnel! They didn't appear as advertised. He thought he flunked his final exam.

I had a similar experience in my encounter with death. Despite forty years of daily spiritual practice, disciplines, prayers, meditation, and many years as a spiritual teacher, I didn't experience any of the signposts of traditional death work. Instead, my death experience had an ordinary, mundane, pedestrian quality.

I laughed at my ignorance in expecting a Hollywood scenario. There were no bells, whistles, or flashing lights. However, there was *something* almost indescribable.

My experience of death went beyond technique or phenomena. The presence I felt was noticeable by its reduced quality and solid universal presence, rather than by its sensory impact. It was noteworthy, in its un-noteworthiness! I had known the presence all my life, but not valued it.

My years of spiritual discipline trained me to discern subtle energies. However, the energy beyond the death bardos was really subtle! It was a background energy, behind events.

Prior to my death experience, I had been in the jaws of death with constant, acute pain for two years. For an additional two years, I battled death daily with chronic pain and continual, acute pain. I was literally more dead than alive. I became intimately familiar with bardo work.

Pain contracts your attention. Jousting with acute pain devoured my entire focus. There was no remaining energy for meditation or spiritual practices. Often, I didn't even have the vital force to "witness" the pain.

In acute pain sieges, the word "God" had no meaning. There was no mental or emotional energy available to conceptualize God.

The quick evaporation of my long-practiced spiritual techniques astonished me. After all the years of work, my precious practices ran for the hills in a flash! Poof! They were gone.

However, something of my altar work remained. Although I couldn't conceptualize God per se, I *remembered* God—as if at a distance or behind a glass wall. Part of me knew God. The direct knowing went beyond mind, beliefs, or concepts. The God Presence was always there, like a Silent Witness.

Behind preoccupying, catastrophic events, part of me felt God's presence. That expanded part of me held a context for my pain. Over time, the space around the pain became my solace.

As I battled death, the pain grew so intense that my identity couldn't contain it. "I" blasted out beyond the pain. I existed in the emptiness surrounding the pain. In this ultimate figure-ground reversal, the emptiness became my new identity, my container.

Like an invisible divine vase, cosmic emptiness held me. The emptiness became more important than my earthly life. Its quiet power and dynamic peace were my refuge from the ravages of pain.

Throughout earthly life, you live under the canopy of your skull. You trot around with your agendas, beliefs, emotions, and identities. There is a second canopy overhead in the arched curve of the earth's atmosphere. It contains the earth's aura, global agendas, and planetary thought forms.

These canopies are unconscious boundaries containing your earthly journey. You don't even notice them—until they disappear. At death, you blast beyond them. Your new container beyond the bardos is infinite, alive emptiness.

The pain I experienced was so powerful that it blew away the canopies. The sides of my house blew off. Like an astronaut with a hole in his spacecraft, I was sucked into the endless vacuum of cosmic night, spinning in infinite space.

The field of nothingness shocked me at first. Its immensity, devoid of definition, disoriented me. Then, I saw my tiny earthly canopies— my skull and the earth's rounded aura—inside the limitless expanse of nothingness. They sat cupped in the hands of God, cradled inside infinite space.

In the magnitude of the Great Immensity, all you can do is surrender. The deconstructed nothingness becomes your ally.

During years of meditation, my knowing of unstructured God Presence had accumulated—one day at a time. I hadn't consciously recognized the Fertile Void then. However, I had banked divine-knowing every time I showed up at my altar. With each consecrated spiritual practice, I made a God deposit. The Divine Energy Bank returned my investment when I most needed it.

My knowing of God was a deep-down, innate connection and trust. The strength of this God-link helped me to endure and triumph over pain. It guided me through the death worlds and back to life.

Buddhists define a good meditation as "Paragate," meaning "Gone beyond." A good meditation is a death experience. It goes beyond earthly life.

Meditative practice helps you die well. Through a lifetime of meditation, I had made friends with the Fertile Void. The Cosmic Dissolve was familiar. Meditation taught me to value the emptiness, rather than fear or dismiss it. My altar work served me well—but not in the way I expected.

The Sufis say there is a presence that neither comes nor goes. That presence is God. That is what you dissolve into at death. That is what you are in life—though you may disqualify it as inconsequential.

Rumi says, when you eventually see through the veils to how things really are, you will keep saying, again and again, "This is not at all how we thought it was!"

The Brink between Life and Death

Life and death, a twisted vine sharing a single root.
—Rabbi Rami M. Shapiro

In your healing journey, you may notice that your spirit hovers between life and death. You may cross back and forth between the worlds, repeatedly. You are trying to evaluate the situation and establish your direction. You may be rehearsing for the other side.

If you decide to pass over, it helps to have friends on the other side or a clear goal to move towards. Sometimes, on the other side you can go to school, take classes with Masters, or do something you really wanted to do in life, but were not able to do. Read Dr. Michael Newton's *Destiny of Souls* and *Journey of Souls* for a clearer picture of life after death.

Having a map of the death journey also helps. At the beginning of your transition, do not be distracted by anything. There may be tumultuous thoughts, stiletto sharp emotions, high velocity buffeting, and turmoil as you traverse the bardos. Make no judgments. Remain a detached witness. Don't hook into their realities. They are illusions.

Keep your focus on the Clear White Light. Some people see it at the end of a long tunnel. If you don't see it, imagine the White Light. If you still can't see it because of darkness and confusion, remember God.

Call upon the angels and your guides to help you find God. The Angels of Death are specially trained to help you. All your allies will help you.

Stay riveted on God. Don't let anything divert your attention. Go into the Light. Soon you will be enraptured, absorbed in God's glorious love. Eventually, you will merge with the Fertile Void, its quiet power, and dynamic peace.

There is hope for glorious God union either way, in life or death— whether you stay to walk with God on earth or become absorbed in

God on the other side. Don't be deceived by thinking that God union only happens through death.

The raptures of God union can be as great while you are in a physical body. In addition, you have the miracle of your physical body with which to enjoy this rare world. Without a body, it can be more difficult to contact loved ones who are still alive.

Don't throw away your physical envelope too quickly. Spiritual escapism can create illusions of the physical plane as impoverished. In addition, escapism can create avoidance of the work you came to do while in a physical body.

Earth is currently one of the richest, most beautiful places in the multiverse. As earth takes its first spiritual initiation, moving from a mundane to a sacred planet, it is one of the most sought-after travel destinations. Crowds of souls await birth certificates. Planetary initiations are rare. It is a privilege to be here now, participating in earth's sacred transformation.

In addition, the joys of earthly life are singular among cosmic travel destinations. Sex, food, emotions, human love, beauty, pleasure, the ability to transmute karma, free will, individuation, variety, drama—these are just a few of the bonuses unique to earthly life. Earth is a rare theme park with many exciting rides not available elsewhere.

Life on the other side offers its own advantages, including the following: freedom, cosmic travel, transcending time/space limits, dropping earth's illusions, release from physical pain and earthly encumbrances, unburdening painful past experiences, understanding the gifts of your pain, understanding your Soul Contract, karma assessments, wisdom trainings, access to Masters and their teachings, renewal, Soul-cluster reunions, a new level of service, and God union.

Is it your time to live or to die? Listen carefully to your Higher Self. Be careful not to escape into a fantasy world. Don't avoid your earthly responsibilities. Pray, "Dear God, show me my highest choice according to your will."

These are deeply personal, important choices. Keep asking questions and listen with a pure and willing heart. Be willing to stay or to leave. Surrender. And you will find your way.

Daily Death and God Union

What if you went through your entire life without realizing
you already have the precious treasure that you are seeking?
—Judith Larkin Reno, Ph. D.

The moment of death is every moment.
—T. S. Eliot

Buddhists say, "If you die before you die, then you don't die when you die." For an easy passage at the end of life, practice dying before you die. Buddhists recommend daily dying. You can use life's many mini-deaths to prepare for Red Foxx's "big one."

In *Stillness Speaks,* spiritual teacher Eckhart Tolle says, "If you can learn to accept and even welcome the endings in your life, you may find that the feeling of emptiness that initially felt uncomfortable turns into a sense of inner spaciousness that is deeply peaceful." Rather than resisting, go into each loss until you find the blessed emptiness. This, essentially, is the death experience. Acceptance of loss, like death, returns you to God.

Both loss and physical death involve ego death. During the death experience, "I" dissolve into God union. I no longer have a separate human self. I merge with blessed emptiness. There is only oneness in God.

This ego death is natural and familiar. You experience it in meditation, in God Ladder aerobics, in the Sacred Now, in sleep, in surrender to loss, and in physical death.

You can make it safe for your ego to die by practicing silence, stopping, conscious breathing, relaxing, smiling, being in the now, witnessing, and meditating. Non-judgmentalness, detachment, humility, selfless giving, and surrender to God's will also dissolve the ego.

Use your God Ladder to train your ego to dissolve into God Source. Practice moving up and down the God Ladder. Consciously focus in your physical body. Then move into your emotions. Move on to your mental body with all its beliefs, concepts, ideology, and thoughts of right and wrong, good and bad. Now, disengage from what you feel physically, emotionally, and mentally.

Move beyond these earthly trappings. Focus your identity in your divine bodies: intuitional, Soul, God Self, and God Source. See your life through the eyes of eternity and infinity. Use your Soul Vision and God Glasses.

This God Ladder calisthenic limbers you up for the trip to God at death. Use your God Ladder to practice detachment and God union. Exercise your spiritual muscles. God Ladder calisthenics increase your spiritual IQ for life's ultimate journey.

With practice, ego death will become familiar, making physical death easier when it comes. Dying is natural. Since you "die" every night when you sleep, how difficult can death be?

Hey! The French call orgasm "le petit mal" or the little death. Orgasm is the moment of God union. Meditators refer to sex as "the poor man's meditation." It is amazing how understanding labels makes the trip to God more fun!

When I merge with God Source, my personal identity becomes obsolete. In its place, I receive God. My identity infinitely expands.

God union is the prize I move toward at death.

Meditation on Death

Find your Light Body Triumphant.
—Judith Larkin Reno, Ph. D.

If you want to know how you will die, notice how you live. Research shows you will die in the same style that you live. Research also shows that anything you do to strengthen your faith in God helps you die well.

Make a decision regarding your relationship with death. See it as an ally. Don't be a victim of death. The following practice meditation helps you die with dignity.

Whenever a life dissolves, a hole in space forms. The Light of God shines through the opening. Tolle says, "The most sacred thing in life is death. That is why the peace of God can come to you through the contemplation and acceptance of death."

When I meditate on my own death, I make friends with it. I consciously take the fear out of it. My death rehearsal smoothes the way. When my time comes, there will be clear, familiar Path to follow.

In my death meditation, I visualize and experience the following.

Meditation on Death

I call upon my Soul and God Self to guide and protect me on my journey through death's gateway. Safe in their hands, I rise above my body. I'm absorbed in a mist of Holy Light.

Radiant Angels of Death lift me higher. Melting my heart with love and joy, they accelerate my vibration. It's a relief to drop the burdens of my body and earthly concerns. Layer after layer of heavy weight falls away.

The Angels of Death guide me to the Vortex of Loving Light. Spinning inside an immense funnel of swarming angels, I ascend through the many worlds to meet God's embrace. We are joyously magnetized Home. There is nothing to do but surrender to the heavenly call.

Surrounded by this shining host, I rise through the Vortex toward God's radiance at its apex. God union is the destination of our Divine Ride.

As I travel through the Vortex of Loving Light, the luminescence hums. I hear a majestic, victorious chorus, much like the Hallelujah Chorus from Handel's Messiah. I hear, "Hallelujah!! Hallelujah!! Rejoice!! God has come. The struggle is over. You are free!!" Flights of angels sing me Home.

Reaching my destination, God's Love is beyond any human experience. In His presence, all judgment and fear drop away. Human agendas disappear, replaced by joyous celebration. Ecstasy and rapture surge through me. Now, beyond words and thought, I dissolve into God's Love. I'm transformed by this Love.

I return to my True Self. I see through eyes of compassion, thrilling at all creation. Awakening from karmic trance, I'm restored to grace and God union. I stand in my Light Body Triumphant.

Resounding like a pure, clear bell, I dwell in peace and joy. I am one with the Vast Sublimity.

Truly, death has no sting—only glory. Use this meditation to practice the way Home.

My favorite description of death comes from the great Sufi poet Hafiz. He says, "The voice of the river that has emptied into the ocean Now laughs and sings just like God."

Verneice Fights Death for Me

There is in the worst of fortunes the best of chances for a happy change.
—Euripides

Rage, rage against the dying of the light.
Do not go softly into that dark night.
—Dylan Thomas

My friend Verneice is a world-class healer. I've seen her heal fevers, infections, and nausea in a few minutes. I've also seen her heal more complex diseases over a longer period of time.

In her sixties, Verneice is a beautiful, full-sized woman with the powers of a Hawaiian kahuna. She is trained as a Taoist priestess. Her eyes are a penetrating, clear blue. They sparkle like a South Sea ocean wave breaking in the sun, spilling out sizzling white foam and dazzling crystals.

Verneice and I had been friends for about twenty years. During that time, she did regular healing treatments for me.

The first time I came home from the hospital, I was weak— like a noodle—from the chemo treatments. It was too painful to lie on Verneice's table. I slumped to the floor for our healing treatment.

I could barely talk from laryngitis. The tremors were so bad, I couldn't hold anything. Black necrotic crust made my legs and feet excruciatingly painful to touch. My dislocated bones and broken vertebra prohibited walking or even turning over without assistance.

Verneice was shaken to see what the disease had done to me. As the healing work progressed, suddenly both Verneice and I heard an eerie, howling sound like wind hurtling down a long corridor.

A large door opened to my left on the inner worlds. I saw the ominous gray wind. It created a horrible sucking sound. Terrified, I knew the Dark Presence wanted to carry me into the Death Worlds.

The menacing sound toyed with me in my vulnerability. My defenselessness fed its appetite. Coming close, it verged on dismembering me. Then suddenly, it mysteriously retreated back into its cavernous den.

Verneice was serious and quiet, assessing the situation. The next time the Deadly Presence stalked me, Verneice was ready for it. On the inner worlds, she raised her generously sized body and thrust it into the doorway.

She hurled the full power of Universal God Force into the face of Death. It was like watching a huge force of nature rise from the ocean floor and strike with precision accuracy. Verneice's tidal wave of energy assaulted the Deadly Presence and stopped its progress.

Verneice continued expanding her energy body until it blocked the doorway. Her impenetrable energy barrier was seamless. Nothing could pass her. She confined the howling hulk with her sheer will and diamond-sharp focus.

Emanating white-hot radiance, she shook her fist in Death's face shouting, "Back off! You're not taking her!"

Staring Death straight in the eye, she said, "You can't have her. She belongs to us. We need her. She's staying right here with us. So, back off!!!"

There was no anger in her voice. Her absolute conviction was a direct line to pure power. Verneice had no fear of Death. She sounded like a mother mandating and corralling an unruly child—rather than a mere mortal commanding the Grim Reaper.

The Deadly Presence sensed the intractable power of Verneice's conviction. The otherworldly wind and weird sucking sound subsided. The door sealed over, as if new skin had grown over it.

When the wind stopped and the Doorway disappeared, I began to cry.

Verneice rocked me in her arms saying, "You're safe. You may be ready to go. You've done your work on earth and you are prepared to pass over. However, we are not ready to let you go. There are too many of us here who love you. We want you with us. We need you.

"I'm not ready for you to go," she confessed.

Verneice fought the enemy with her bare fists, words, and spitfire energy. Her naturalness in the face of Death was awesome. Where I didn't have strength to fight for my life, Verneice stood up and fought for me. She saved my life. She was my champion.

"I love you Verneice. Thank you! Thank you! You saved my life."

We lay on the floor with our arms around each other, like little kids on a camp-out looking at the night stars. Pure golden Love Light energy filled the room.

Verneice changed my life forever. With matter-of-fact dominion, she performed a miracle.

God works in wondrous ways!

DON'T JUDGE

By yielding you may obtain victory.
—Unknown

Take not gain or loss to heart.
Undertakings bring good fortune.
Everything serves to further.
—Confucius

Maybe So, Maybe Not

There are two tragedies in life. One is not getting what you want.
The other is getting what you want.
—Oscar Wilde

In the roller coaster ride of medical procedures, tests, diagnoses, and prognoses, I looked for inner stability. Every day contained life-and-death decisions. There were many crises. I tended to catastrophize each one. However, if I gave my energy to panic and anxiety, I had less energy for healing.

Over time, I learned that apparent tragedy always worked itself out. Problems eventually got resolved. I solved one problem at a time, even if the solution required radical adaptation and new coping skills.

I could have saved myself the earlier worry. The truth is God's in charge of each outcome. I just had to show up with the right attitude of openness and non-judgmentalness.

The following story, from an East Indian spiritual tradition, helped me gain a stable perspective in the midst of trouble.

Once there was a farmer, whose son broke his leg. The locals said, "What a misfortune." The farmer replied, "Maybe so. Maybe not."

The next week, the army came to conscript young men. Because the son's leg was broken, he was not taken. The neighbors said, "What a boon! How lucky you are!" The farmer replied, "Maybe so. Maybe not."

The following week, the farmer's horse jumped the fence and ran away. Because the son's leg was broken, he couldn't catch the horse. The locals said, "What a misfortune." The farmer replied, "Maybe so. Maybe not."

The next month, the farmer's horse returned home, bringing twelve wild horses with him. The neighbors said, "What a boon." The farmer said, "Maybe so. Maybe not."

I think of this story when I'm in the midst of apparent tragedy, crisis, and negative events. It restores my equanimity.

Make No Judgments

Everything has its wonders, even darkness and silence.
—Helen Keller

"Avoid judgment" is a basic premise of spiritual training. My Guides often said, "When you think you are doing your best work, we don't necessarily see it as all that great. On the other hand, when you think you are doing your worst work, we often see it as triumphant and heroic!"

Remember the differences between judgment and discernment. Discernment is clear perceiving. It is objective, unattached assessment without excessive emotionality, moral charge, or polarization. Discernment is naming without blaming.

Discernment is an ally. Judgment is an enemy.

Especially, avoid judging yourself wrong for your disease. You are responsible for creating events from the divine levels of your Soul

Contract and God union. However, these levels can be hidden from earthly eyes.

Honor your earthly level. Be gentle with it and nurture it. Use your responsibility as power to change, not power to blame or call yourself wrong. You did nothing wrong regarding your medical condition. God is not punishing you through illness.

You can get unproductively lost in the blaming question, "Why me, God?" Instead, start from the assumption that God did it right. Then, you automatically move into a creative universe.

Avoid spiritual circles that cast judgment against sickness. Their assumption is that you did something wrong if you get sick. If you just correct a bad thought or two—voila—you would never would get ill.

The Truth is, the healthy are no "better" than the sick. Saints die of illness every day of the week—many from cancer. You are not a bad girl/boy if you get sick. Illness is often far more complex than simple solutions imply—especially for spiritual initiates.

Spiritual pathwork is rigorous. Trials abound in spiritual life. The lives of saints portray crucifixion, stake burnings, poverty, Job initiations, tremendous loss, tribulation, and illness.

Testing the spiritual initiate is comparable to tempering the steel to make the sword strong for battle. The spiritual gifts of these difficult passages are enormous. Deeper initiation, wisdom, love, and intimacy with God are the harvest.

Don't be deceived by illness. All illness is part of God's plan. Much more benefit may be accruing than meets the eye—or mind! Illness may be essential to your spiritual initiation.

In addition, you may be healing the collective. By taking on illness, the initiate can save lives, by-pass global suffering, and accelerate human evolution.

For example, since we all are one, if one person cycles-up through pain, everyone benefits. The higher vibration enters the collective Pool of Luminosity. These powerful healing energies transform and evolve human DNA.

Frequently in the East, masters carry the negative karma of their students. The guru is called the "darkness eater." The master may transmute his student's karma through his own physical illness.

Pictures of Herakhan Babaji show his belly so distended that he looks pregnant. When asked about his appearance, he said he was taking his students' pain to liberate them.

Sometimes in families, one person carries the pain for the group. The entire family may transform through one member's illness. Indeed, one person's illness affects everyone that person knows. It can focus and elevate friends, family, and acquaintances.

In addition to spiritual initiation and planetary service, there are other reasons a Soul might choose physical illness. Through a positive approach to pain, you can dissolve past-life karma and reach liberation. You can accelerate your spiritual growth.

Numerologically, if you are in a number 9 incarnation, through illness you may be completing thousands of previous lifetimes, resolving old conflicts, forgiving ignorance, and transcending the past. Transmutation through personal pain can create closure and provide a great final triumph.

Occasionally, a spiritual initiate transmutes a destructive weather pattern or regional catastrophe through illness. The initiate's sacrifice can protect and improve large numbers of lives.

For example, prior to the Russian nuclear disaster at Chernobyl during the 1980's, several of my spiritual-path students dreamed about the disaster—months before its occurrence. These students knew nothing of each other. However, their dreams were similar.

Their dreams involved flying above Chernobyl, rescuing children and families long before the catastrophe. Transcending the time/space box, initiates rehearsed, comforted, and prepared families to cope with impending disaster. They actually created solutions before the problem occurred on earth.

Some initiates contracted colds during this period. They complained that they were so busy—working all night in their sacred dream assignments—that their bodies were exhausted.

However, their illness was a small price to pay for the service they provided to humanity. The initiate's sacrifice was part of a larger planetary plan.

Ancient wisdom says, "It is a great boon to do sacrificial work for the tribe." There is no judgment or blame toward a sick person.

Rather, there is honor for his courage. The tribe respects his service in transmuting darkness to Light through illness. The tribe elevates and esteems the sick person for his consecration.

Illness can be a path of purification for oneself and the collective.

The path of pain is often called "the fast path" of spiritual growth. It is only available to willing and devoted servants of God.

Milarepa's House

> *The basic difference between an ordinary man and a warrior*
> *is that a warrior takes everything as a challenge, while and*
> *ordinary man takes everything either as a blessing or a curse.*
> —Don Juan, Carlos Castaneda's Teacher

Milarepa was a famous Tibetan master. One day a monk came to him and said, "Teach me, Dear Master, how I might become like you. I desire to be enlightened and free."

Milarepa said to the aspiring monk, "Go to the field and build a house."

The student wondered what house construction had to do with enlightenment. However, he had learned to trust the outlandish requests of enlightened beings. As eccentric as they appear, in the end they reveal truth.

The student was eager for growth. He had been on the Path for many years and still had not attained liberation. Highly motivated for a breakthrough, he set off to build a house.

House construction was not easy. The winters were long in the mountains, with up to one hundred feet of snow on the roof. In their remote location, it was difficult to obtain building materials. There was no one to help him.

Nevertheless, the monk persevered. After eighteen months, he finished the house. Proud of his accomplishment and anticipating his enlightenment rewards, he ran to Milarepa to tell him the good news.

Milarepa listened and said, "Good. Now, go and tear the house down."

"What!" said the shocked monk in disbelief. "It took months of hard labor to get this far. I thought my reward would be enlightenment."

"If you want enlightenment, go tear the house down," Milarepa replied.

Shaking his head, the monk returned to his beautiful, new house. He sat there for many days, stunned and cold in his heart. He felt betrayed and hurt.

However, he couldn't deny that he still desired enlightenment more than anything in the world. He felt sure Milarepa had the answer he was seeking. After all, Milarepa was a famous master. He must have a plan behind his outrageous demands.

After several weeks, the monk slowly began tearing down the house. At first, his heart wasn't in it. Gradually, as the work progressed, he lost his anger toward Milarepa. He began thinking, "That sly dog. I bet this exercise in destruction is a test to see how much I want enlightenment. I'm going to finish this job and go claim my prize. I'll fix him. Won't Milarepa be surprised!"

The monk finished tearing down the house. Proud of his accomplishment, he ran to Milarepa with the good news. Milarepa listened and said, "Very good. Now, I want you to go back and build another house in the same spot."

"What!" said the monk in amazement. "First, I build the house that you request. At great energy and expense to myself, I might add! Then, I surrender to your inane request to tear the house down, thinking you are testing my love for enlightenment. I thought my reward for following your instructions would be the enlightenment I so deeply desire."

"If you truly want enlightenment, you must go build another house," was the Master's reply.

Exhausted and confused, the monk returned to the land. He had to re-evaluate his life and think deeply. He had suffered greatly so far. Why should he continue following these non-productive instructions?

As the days passed, nothing satisfied him. Only his love for God union and enlightenment persisted.

He could not stop thinking about his Master. He knew the Master had the information he was seeking. Why didn't the Master just tell him the answer and get on with it? Why be sidetracked by house construction? He wanted enlightenment, not another house.

Disgruntled and muttering under his breath, the monk began building another house for the Master. This time it took a year of hard work. It went faster since he knew the job better and he still had some materials left from the last house.

By the end of the year, he had reconciled himself that spiritual masters were crazy. To get enlightened he'd just have to put up with irrational requests. After all, some enlightened masters ran naked through the village. They had glazed eyes and matted hair. They never washed. At least Milarepa wasn't asking him to do that!

When the second house was finished, the monk went to his Master. Again, he was expecting a reward for his hard work and obedience. But again, Milarepa told the monk to go back and tear the house down.

Numbed and staggering, the monk began hacking away at the house he had so lovingly built for his Master. This time he didn't care why Milarepa had said to destroy the house. All he could see was his love for God and his determination to become enlightened like his Master.

Once again, after the house was destroyed, Milarepa sent the monk back to construct another house. This cycle of building and destroying continued for another ten years. By then, the monk's heart was singing and he reached enlightenment. He was liberated from judgment.

He had learned to dwell in surrender and the merging.

TREASURE

The spiritual path wrecks the body—
And afterwards restores it to health.
It destroys the house to unearth the treasure.
—Jellaludin Rumi

Cycles, Paradox, and Diamonds

Find your indestructible, adamantine diamond spirit.
—Judith Larkin Reno, Ph. D.

Life and death are natural cycles of earth's duality—construction and de-construction. If you live long enough, you experience both tragedy and triumph. Like Milarepa's house, God continuously destroys earthly life to make way for new creation.

The cycles of earthly life are not personal. Fluctuation is the nature of duality inside the time/space box. If you get in the swing of accepting earthly cycles, you save yourself suffering.

With catastrophic illness, the opposites manifest in a unique way. You fight to live against a backdrop of surrender to God's will. The opposites of fighting and surrendering coexist within you. The cycles of construction and deconstruction are not sequential, but simultaneous! Creating this paradoxical house of healing is far more complicated than Milarepa's assignment.

Illness teaches acceptance of cycles and paradox. By holding the cognitive dissonance of paradox, you discover many paths to Truth. With paradox, the mind and spirit stay fluid. The capacity to contain opposites increases your spiritual IQ, your enlightenment, and your healing.

Illness also teaches that the great treasure you are seeking lies within you. Through illness, you discover your True Identity, extending far beyond earthly house-building. Endless house-building is the way of the world. Your True Identity transcends earthly conventions.

In the midst of external chaos, illness teaches you to anchor in your internal, permanent, indestructible, adamantine diamond core. Beyond earthly cycles of life and death, your ultimate treasure is your God union.

Honor the Opposites

When I see that I am nothing, that is wisdom. When I see that I am everything, that is love. Between these two my life moves.
—Sri Nisargadatta

Ancient Buddhist wisdom says, "The wise man walks in both worlds." In the healing journey, your consciousness expands to include the opposites of your earthly and divine natures. Through the spiritual initiation of illness, you learn to honor both worlds: facts and Truth, your personal will and God's will.

The God Ladder teaches you to embrace this ultimate duality: your earthly and divine natures. You serve both the passing and the permanent, the ephemeral and eternal, your body and spirit.

Eventually, you accept that opposites co-exist in human life. Rather than polarize into "either/or," you live according to the ultimate paradox of "both/and." Your earthly and divine natures inform each other. You serve both their needs appropriately.

However, your mind says, "How can opposites exist in the same space and time?" "How can I contain the yes and the no, simultaneously?" "How can my earthly and divine natures live in harmony?" "How can I fight to live and surrender to death, simultaneously?" "How can I say yes to both life and death?"

The great paradox of containing the opposites cannot be solved with your mind. Mind is not up to the task. Comfort with paradox demands spiritual IQ. Your spiritual intelligence reflects your capacity to contain ambiguity, uncertainty, and opposites. Illness opens you to the Great Mystery and accepting paradox.

Helen Keller says, "To keep our faces toward change and behave like free spirits in the presence of fate is strength undefeatable." Both your earthly and divine natures are your birthright.

Traveling the God Ladder integrates your earthly and divine bodies. Resolving the dualities of illness, you move into wholeness and healing—whether it is spiritual or physical healing.

When you honor both earthly and divine realities, you deny neither, fluidly traveling between both worlds. Idealism coexists with earthly realism. You embrace both the absolute and the relative worlds, giving each its place.

With earthly birth, you access a time/space corridor—call it your life. Your divine Soul Contract predetermines the events of your life. However, within the earthly time/space box, you must act as if you have free will. Both destiny and free will coexist.

Your human life fulfills the laws of destiny until its karma exhausts. You might as well develop a strong divine witness point and enjoy the show until events finish unspooling! Acceptance of divine will is a key to victory.

Simultaneously, at the earthly level, struggle with all your personal will to do what is right. This way you can't lose. You satisfy both your earthly and divine natures.

To honor the opposites, don't be attached to outcomes. And above all, make no judgments.

Pain and illness force you to transcend your limited earth-bound identity to explore your True Self. Illness insists that you become large enough to embrace the opposites of your earthly and divine natures.

Enlightenment

> *Enlightenment is the ego's biggest disappointment.*
> —Chogyam Trungpa Rinpoche, Buddhist

The following wisdom teachings often unfold on the spiritual path of illness. They lead to your internal God treasure and enlightenment.

- Enlightenment is not a flashy experience.—Maharishi Mahesh Yogi
- Before enlightenment, chop wood and carry water. After enlightenment, chop wood and carry water.—Buddhist
- After the ecstasy, the laundry.—Jack Kornfield
- Enlightenment is knowing that everything is as it should be—accepting what is.—Judith Larkin Reno, Ph. D.
- Enlightenment is a grief experience. It is the death of one illusion after another.—Judith Larkin Reno, Ph. D.
- Enlightenment is surfing the chaos of life without ego expectation to change it. Rather, enjoying the ride.—Judith Larkin Reno, Ph. D.
- There's nothing to do but rejoice and give thanks!—Judith Larkin Reno, Ph. D.
- Enlightenment means you've run out of questions.—Frederick Lenz, Ph. D.
- Enlightenment is taking back your projections.—Yudhishtara
- Your personal God concept is the collection of your highest and best illusions at any given moment.—Judith Larkin Reno, Ph. D.
- Everyone gets the God he deserves.—Judith Larkin Reno, Ph. D.
- There is only one Truth in my church. So far I'm the only member.—Thomas Carlisle
- All paths lead nowhere.—Carlos Castaneda
- The Truth is a pathless land.—Krishnamurti
- Thought clouds.—Bernie Gunther, Ph. D.
- There is no other way. Every time the mind goes astray, bring it back to Source.—Sri Ramana Maharshi
- Enlightenment is to rise above thinking and disidentify with thought.—Eckhart Tolle
- Understanding is the booby prize.—Werner Erhardt
- The mind must recognize and penetrate its own state of being, not being this or that, here or there, then or now, but just timeless being.—Sri Nisargadatta
- Enlightenment is to rise above suffering.—Buddha
- Be melting snow.—Rumi

Treasure

The silent hand poured holy rivers of Love all over me.
—Judith Larkin Reno, Ph. D.

I'm profoundly grateful that I can feel God's love. Where does all this love between God and me come from? Nothing has destroyed it through all of life's ups and downs. Instead, it keeps growing! The God Presence inside never leaves.

To know God and feel God's love is the greatest treasure. Indeed, "the treasure lies deep" within. Illness can help you find the treasure.

Blessings in your dances with elephants. May you dance the dream awake. May you discover the great treasure of God union within you. May you find your adamantine diamond spirit.

Ganesha is the Hindu elephant deity of good luck and treasure. May all the elephants in your tent transform to Ganeshas!

RECOMMENDED RESOURCES

Audio Tapes

Pema Chodron Tapes. Robert and Jill Walker, 330 E. Van Hoesen, Portage, MI 49002. Phone: 269-384-4167. E-mail: *gtapes@aol.com.*

Gangaji Pain Tapes. The Gangaji Foundation, 505-A San Marin Dr. Ste 120, Novato, CA 94945. Phone: 1-800-267-9205. Internet address: *www. gangaji.org.*

Thich Nhat Hahn Tapes. Great Path Tapes & Books. Internet address: *www.seaox. com/thich.html.*

Stephen Levine Pain Tapes. Warm Rock Tapes, PO Box 100, Chamisal, NM 87521. Internet address: *www.gillmacmillan.*

Belleruth Naparstek. *For People with Cancer.* Time Warner Audio Books. 1-800-800-8661.

Dr. Judith Larkin Reno Tapes on Healing and Meditation. Gateway University, 1698 Crystal Ridge Court, Vista, CA 92081. Internet address: *dr.reno@att.net.*

Dr. Carl Simonton. *Getting Well.* NY, NY: St. Martin's Press Audio Renaissance Tapes, 1987.

Eckhart Tolle Pain Tapes. Phone: 866-544-7611. Internet address: *www.store. yahoo.com/onlinesuccessbroker.*

Bibliography

Albom, Mitch. *Tuesdays with Morrie.* NY, NY: Doubleday Publishers, 1997.

Armstrong, Lance. *It's Not About the Bike: My Journey Back to Life.* NY, NY: Penguin Putnam, 2000.

Assagioli, Roberto. *Psychosynthesis: A Manual of Principles and Techniques.* NY, NY: Viking Press, 1971.

Bailey, Alice. *Esoteric Healing.* NY, NY: Lucis Publishing, 1953.

Balsekar, Ramesh. *Consciousness Speaks.* Redondo Beach, CA: Advaita Press, 1992.

Barks, Coleman. *The Essential Rumi.* San Francisco, CA: Harper Collins Publishers, 1995.

————. *Delicious Laughter: Rambunctious Teaching Stories from the Mathnawi Rumi.* Athens, GA: Maypop, 1990.

————, & John Moyne. *Say I Am You: Rumi.* Athens, GA: Maypop, 1994.

Becker, Robert, & Gary Sheldon. *The Body Electric: Electromagnetism and the Foundation of Life.* NY, NY: William Morrow, 1985.

Benson, Herbert. *The Mind-Body Effect.* NY, NY: Simon and Schuster, 1979.

Bolen, Jean Shinoda. *Close to the Bone: Life-Threatening Illness and the Search for Meaning.* NY, NY: Simon & Schuster Touchstone, 1996.

Borysenko, Joan. *A Woman's Book of Life: The Biology, Psychology, and Spirituality of the Feminine Life Cycle.* NY, NY: Riverhead Books, 1996.

Bradshaw, John. *Healing the Shame That Binds You.* Deerfield Beach, FL: Health Communications, 1988.

Breathnach, Sarah. *Simple Abundance.* NY, NY: Time Warner, 1995.

Brennan, Barbara Ann. *Hands of Light.* NY, NY: *Bantam,* 1988.

Bruyere, Rosalyn. *Wheels of Light: A Study of the Chakras.* Arcadia, CA: Bon Productions, 1989.

Burns, David D. *The Feeling Good Handbook.* NY, NY: Plume Books of Penguin, 1989.

Campbell, Joseph. *The Power of the Myth.* NY, NY: Doubleday, 1988.

Canfield, Jack, & Mark Victor Hansen. *Chicken Soup for the Soul.* Deerfield Beach, FL: Health Communications, 1993.

————. *Chicken Soup for the Surviving Soul.* 1996.

Catalano, Ellen, & Kimeron Hardin. *The Chronic Pain Control Workbook.* Oakland, CA: New Harbinger, 1996.

Caudill, Margaret. *Managing Pain Before It Manages You.* NY, NY: Guilford Press, 1995.

Chodron, Pema. *Start Where You Are: A Guide to Compassionate Living.* NY, NY: Shambala Press, 1994.

Chopra, Deepak. *Quantum Healing: Exploring the Frontiers of Mind/Body Medicine.* NY, NY: Bantam, 1989.

———. *Ageless Body, Timeless Mind: The Quantum Alternative to Growing Old.* NY, NY: Harmony Books, 1993.

———. *The Seven Spiritual Laws of Success.* San Rafael, CA: Amber-Allen Publishing, 1994.

Cota-Robles, Patricia Diane. *The Awakening . . . Eternal Youth, Vibrant Health, Radiant Beauty.* Tucson, AZ: The New Age Study of Humanity's Purpose, 1993.

———. *The Next Step.* 1989.

———. *Take Charge of Your Life.* 1983.

Cousins, Norman. *Anatomy of an Illness as Perceived by the Patient.* NY, NY: Bantam, 1981.

Dossey, Larry. *Space, Time, and Medicine.* Boulder, CO: Shambhala, 1982.

Dychtwald, Ken. *Bodymind.* NY, NY: Tarcher/Putnam Books, 1977.

Dyer, Wayne. *Real Magic: Creating Miracles in Everyday Life.* NY, NY: Harper Collins Publishers, 1992.

Evans-Wentz, W. Y. *The Tibetan Book of the Dead.* NY, NY: Oxford University Press, 1960.

Feinstein, David, & Stanley Krippner. *Personal Mythology: Using Ritual, Dreams, and Imagination to Discover Your Inner Story.* Los Angeles, CA: Jeremy Tarcher Inc., 1988.

Gangaji. *You Are That, Volume 1.* Boulder, CO: Satsang Press, 1995.

———. *You Are That, Volume 2.* 1996.

Gawain, Shakti. *Living in the Light.* San Rafael, CA: New World Library, 1986.

Geffen, Jeremy. *The Journey Through Cancer: An Oncologist's Seven-Level Program for Healing and Transforming the Whole Person.* NY, NY: Random House, 2000.

Gerber, Richard, M. D. *Vibrational Medicine.* Santa Fe, NM: Bear, 1988.

Gibran, Kahlil. *The Prophet.* NY, NY: Alfred Knopf, 1965.

Gold, E. J. *The American Book of the Dead.* San Francisco, CA: And/Or Press, 1975.

Godman, David. *Be As You Are: The Teachings of Sri Ramana Maharshi.* Boston, MA: Arkana, 1985.

Godman, David. *Papaji: Interview.* Boulder, CO: Avadhuta Foundation, 1993.

Grey, Alex. *Sacred Mirrors.* Rochester, VT: Inner Traditions International, 1990.

Hanh, Thich Nhat. *Teachings on Love.* Berkeley, CA: Parallax Press, 1997.

_____. *The Sun My Heart.* 1988.

_____. *Zen Keys.* NY, NY: Doubleday, 1974.

_____. *The Miracle of Mindfulness: A Manual on Meditation.*

Harvey, Andrew. *The Way of Passion: A Celebration of Rumi.* Berkeley, CA: Frog, Ltd., 1994.

Hay, Louise. *You Can Heal Your Life.* Santa Monica, CA: Hay House, 1982.

Holmes, Ernest. *The Basic Ideas of Science of Mind.* Marina del Rey, CA: De Vorss, 1957.

Hurnard, Hannah. *Mountains of Spices.* Wheaton, IL: Tyndale House Publishers, 1977.

_____. *Hinds' Feet on High Places.*

Kabat-Zinn, Jon. *Wherever You Go, There You Are: Mindfulness Meditation.* NY, NY: Hyperion, 1994.

King, Dean & Jessica, & Jonathan Pearlroth. *Cancer Combat: Cancer Survivors Share Their Guerrilla Tactics to Help You Win the Fight of Your Life.* NY, NY: Bantam Books, 1998.

Krieger, Dolores. *The Therapeutic Touch: How to Use Your Hands to Help Or Heal.* Englewood Cliffs, NJ: Prentice-Hall, 1979.

Ladinsky, Daniel. *The Gift: Poems by Hafiz.* NY, NY: Penguin Books, 1999.

_____ *I Heard God Laughing: Renderings of Hafiz.* Walnut Creek, CA: Sufism Reoriented, 1996.

_____. *The Subject Tonight is Love: Sixty Wild and Sweet Poems of Hafiz.* North Myrtle Beach, SC: Pumpkin House, 1996.

Laskow, Leonard. *Healing With Love.* San Francisco, CA: Harper Collins, 1992.

LeShan, Lawrence. *Cancer as a Turning Point: A Handbook for People with Cancer, Their Families, and Health Professionals.* NY, NY: Penguin Putnam, 1994.

Lowen, Alexander. *The Language of the Body*. NY, NY: Macmillan, 1958.

Levine, Stephen. *Healing into Life and Death*. NY, NY: Doubleday Anchor Books, 1987.

————. *A Gradual Awakening*.

————. *Meetings at the Edge*.

————. *Who Dies?*

Marooney, Kimberly. *Angel Blessings*. Carmel, CA: Merrill-West, 1995.

————. *The Seven Gifts of Your Guardian Angel*. Gloucester, MA: Fair Winds Press, 2003.

————. *Angel Love*. 2004.

Milanovich, Norma. *The Light Shall Set You Free*. Albuquerque, NM: Athena Publishing, 1996.

Milewski, John, & Virginia Harford. *The Crystal Sourcebook*. Sedona, AZ: Mystic Crystal Publications, 1987.

Motoyama, Hiroshi. *Theories of the Chakras*. Wheaton, IL: Quest, 1981.

Murphy, Joseph. *The Power of Your Subconscious Mind*. NY, NY: Bantam Books, 1963.

Myss, Caroline. *Anatomy of the Spirit: The Seven Stages of Power and Healing*. NY, NY: Harmony Books, 1996.

Nadeem, Satyam. *From Onions To Pearls*. Carlsbad, CA: Hay House, 1996.

Newton, Michael. *Destiny of Souls: New Case Studies of Life between Lives*. St. Paul, MN: Llewellyn Publications, 2002.

————. *Journey of Souls: Case Studies of Life between Lives*. St. Paul, MN: Llewellyn Publications, 2002.

Sri Nisargadatta Maharaj. *I Am That*. Durham, NC: Acorn Press, 1973.

Northrup, Christiane. *Women's Bodies, Women's Wisdom*. NY, NY: Bantam, 1995.

Osborne, Arthur. *Ramana Maharshi and the Path of Self Knowledge*. York Beach, ME: Samuel Weiser, 1970.

Pearsall, Paul. *Making Miracles*. NY, NY: Avon Books, 1991.

Pelletier, Kenneth R. *Mind as Healer, Mind as Slayer*. NY, NY: Delacorte, 1977.

Piper, Watty, *The Little Engine That Could*. NY, NY: Grosset & Dunlap, 1986.

Ponder, Catherine. *The Healing Secret of the Ages*. West Nyack, NY, NY: Parker Publishing, 1967.

_____. *Open Your Mind to Receive.* Marina del Rey, CA: DeVorss, 1983.

Quinly, Cariel. *Crop Circle Cards: The Living Oracle.* Vista, CA: Cosmic Connections, 1998.

Ram Dass. *Journey of Awakening: A Meditator's Guidebook.* NY, NY: Bantam Books, 1990.

_____. *Still Here: Embracing Aging, Changing, and Dying.* NY, NY: Penguin Putnam Riverhead Books, 2000.

_____. *Be Here Now.*

Remen, Naomi. *Kitchen Table Wisdom.* NY, NY: Riverhead Books, 1996.

Reno, Judith Larkin. *A Mystic's View of War: Using the God Ladder for Clarity.* Philadelphia, PA: Xlibris, 2002.

Robbins, Anthony. *Awaken the Giant Within.* NY, NY: Simon Schuster, 1991.

Rodegast, Pat, & Judith Stanton. *Emmanuel's Book.* NY, NY: Bantam Books, 1985.

Roberts, Elizabeth, & Elias Amidon. *Earth Prayers.* San Francisco, CA: Harper Collins Publishers, 1991.

Rosenberg, Larry. *Living in the Light of Death: On the Art of Being Truly Alive.* Boston, MA: Shambhala, 2000.

Subramuniyaswami, Satguru Sivaya. *Loving Ganesha: Hinduism's Endearing Elephant-Faced God.* USA/India: Himalayan Academy, 2000. (Contact Saiva Siddhanta Yoga Order, Kapaa, HI).

Saint-Exupery, Antoine de. *The Little Prince.* NY, NY: Harcourt Brace Jovanovich, 1971.

Silva, Jose. *The Silva Mind Control Method of Mental Dynamics.* NY, NY: Pocket Books, 1988.

Schwartz, Jack. *Voluntary Controls: Exercises for Creative Meditation and for Activating the Potential of the Chakras.* NY, NY: Dutton, 1978.

Sherman, Harold. *How to Make ESP Work For You.* NY, NY: Ballantine Books, 1964.

Shealy, Norman. *The Pain Game.* Berkeley, CA: Celestial Arts, 1976.

Sheldon, Mary. *Guidance from the Darkness: The Transforming Power of the Divine Feminine in Difficult Times.* NY, NY: Jeremy Tarcher Putnam, 2000.

Siegel, Bernie S. *Love, Medicine and Miracles.* NY, NY: Harper and Row, 1986.

Simonton, O. Carl, Stephanie Matthews Simonton, & James Creighton. *Getting Well Again.* Los Angeles, CA: J.P. Tarcher, 1978.

Sogyal Rinpoche. *The Tibetan Book of Living and Dying.* NY, NY: HarperCollins, 1993.

Spalding, Baird. *Life and Teaching of the Masters of the Far East,* 5 Volumes. Marina del Rey, CA: De Vorss and Company, 1924.

Stone, Joshua. *The Ascended Masters Light the Way, Vol. 5.* Sedona, AZ: Light Technology Publishing, 1995.

Tate, David. *Health, Hope & Healing.* NY, NY: M. Evans & Company, 1989.

Tolle, Eckhart. *The Power of Now: A Guide to Spiritual Enlightenment.* Novato, CA: New World Library, 1999.

Trott, Susan. *The Holy Man.* NY, NY: Riverhead Books, 1997.

_____. *The Holy Man's Journey.*

Walsch, Neale Donald. *Conversations with God, Book 1.* N.Y.: Putnam, 1995.

_____. *Conversations with God, Book 2,* Charlottesville, VA: Hampton Roads, 1995.

Weil, Andrew. *Natural Health, Natural Medicine.* Boston, MA: Houghton Mifflin, 1990

Wilber, Ken. *Grace and Grit: Spirituality and Healing in the Life and Death of Treya Killam Wilber.* Boston, MA: Shambala, 1993.

Wolf, Fred Alan. *The Body Quantum.* NY, NY: Macmillan, 1986.

Wulfing, Sulamith. *Angels Great and Small.* Amsterdam: V.O.C., 1981.

Yogananda, Paramahansa. *Autobiography of a Yogi.* Los Angeles, CA: Self Realization Fellowship, 1993.

Films

The Barbarian Invasions. This fine Canadian film explores end-of-life choices. Modern medical care is one of the barbarians in this refreshing look at compassionate dying. Modern dying triggers difficult issues, such as father-son alienation, fragmented families, coming to terms with ignoble aspects of your nature, assigning meaning to your life, dealing with pain, and reconciling values differences with someone you love.

Behind the Red Door. Kiefer Sutherland, Kyra Sedgwick, and Stockard Channing star in this story of a brother and sister entwined in dark family secrets. As Kyra helps Kiefer die, the two are redeemed and spiritually healed.

Castaways. As the lone survivor of a plane crash, Tom Hanks' character makes it to a deserted island. His survival skills are those of the healing journey. A catastrophic life event is isolative and demolishing. The life skills Hanks demonstrates are a play book for reconstructing a destroyed life and re-entering normalcy.

Educating Rita. Michael Caine stars in this film showing the determination and grit it takes to move from one world into another, which describes the healing journey. Healing is similar to Rita's journey, breaking out of a lower class and entering a higher, educated class. Healing requires thresholding liminalities to break free from one reality and penetrate another.

Fierce Grace. Our national treasure and a lifetime spiritual teacher, Ram Dass describes his bout with death and surviving catastrophic illness, as he recuperates from a stroke.

Healing and Dying. Stephen Levine. Reel.com.

Healing and the Mind. Bill Moyers. Reel.com.

Healing and the Unconscious. Reel.com.

Healing from Within. Reel.com.

Healing Spirit. Featuring Dr. Deepak Chopra and Dr. Bernie Siegel. Reel.com.

My Life as a House. Kevin Kline's character faces terminal illness and awakens to his lifetime avoidance of intimacy. His new awareness creates a rich new life with friends and family.

My Life Without Me. A young woman in her twenties faces dying of cancer in her unique way, leaving audio tapes to her two young children for each birthday up to 21.

Spontaneous Healing. Dr. Andrew Weil. Yahoo.com.

The Sleepy Time Gal. Jacqueline Bisset stars in this intimate story of a woman with a vagabond Soul Contract. She marches to her own drummer, both in her unusual life and in dealing with her death.

Tuesdays with Morrie. Based on Mitch Albom's book, this film, produced by Oprah Winfry and starring Jack Lemon, shows a student following his esteemed professor's journey as he approaches death with rare insight and nourishing wisdom to share.

Wit. Oscar winning Emma Thompson stars in this hard-hitting film revealing the heroic struggle of battling cancer. Excellently directed by Mike Nichols, with a first-rate script based on Margaret Edson's book.

Products

Rev. Maggie Smith's Hope Spray shifts the subtle energies in the room from sadness to hope. It can pull you out of a negative hole, restoring your hope, even when the doctors aren't offering any. Rev. Maggie is a Gateway Minister whose flower essences and aroma therapy change the etheric plane to support your healing. They really work! Call her at Flower Essence Energy: 1-800-213-7484.